# Beyond Training

# Beyond Training

## Mastering the Art of
## Contemporary Medicine

*Kevin P. Glynn, M.D.*

Writer's Showcase
presented by *Writer's Digest*
San Jose  New York  Lincoln  Shanghai

Beyond Training
Mastering the Art of Contemporary Medicine

Writer's Showcase
presented by *Writer's Digest*
an imprint of iUniverse.com, Inc.

For information address:
iUniverse.com, Inc.
620 North 48th Street, Suite 201
Lincoln, NE 68504-3467
www.iuniverse.com

ISBN: 0-595-13493-9

Printed in the United States of America

# Contents

# *Preface*

Recently in our community an accomplished and respected doctor despaired over the compromises imposed by contemporary practice. He drove home in the middle of the day, selected a revolver from his gun collection, and shot a bullet through his head. Dismayed colleagues recognized him as the latest casualty in the war between concerned physicians and medicine for profit.

While this case is extreme it is a true story. Doctors and nurses struggle daily as they try to practice competent medicine when everyone is impatient and technology overrides compassion.

Medical school applications are as robust as ever, yet practicing physicians' morale is at a low ebb. Nurses are leaving the bedside for less stressful jobs. Patients vibrate in a gridlock of unfulfilled expectations. Values seemingly essential to professional identity are under barrage. Is the integrity of the healing arts at stake?

This book aims to restore the confidence and power to help the sick. The ideas Harry the young physician learns from his mentors will help others grow beyond the limits of training and master the art of contemporary medicine.

Kevin Glynn, M. D.

# Chapter 1.

# Trouble with Harry

**O**nce upon a time there was a young doctor named Harry. His formal name was Abner Harrison Humbleton, but he didn't like his first name, and his initials sounded like someone sneezing. So he preferred to be called Harry. Harry was a good doctor, respected by his colleagues, appreciated by his patients, and loved by his family. He worked hard to heal all those who came to him for help.

Harry's background suited his destiny as a physician. He was the oldest child in his family, with all the resultant strivings and insecurities bred into his personality. His father was a lawyer, and his mother taught history before she married. From the time he was twelve years old Harry knew he would go into a profession. Bright and conforming, he performed well in school. He reasoned that if he did what the teachers asked, he would get the most benefit from the courses, and would get good grades as well.

Harry was dark, with curly black hair that constantly fell over his forehead. His face was querulous and he walked with an ambling shuffle that hid his anxieties. By his junior year in high school he reached six feet tall and weighed two hundred pounds. Though primarily a student, he went out for football because he thought it was the thing to do. He could move moderately fast, but he was gentle and so spent most of his time as a bench warmer. The coach lamented that if Harry was a little meaner, he could have been a good football player.

But for Harry, playing sports was a way to be with others. He liked to win, but didn't like having to inflict pain in order to prevail. If the team lost, he would be disappointed, but couldn't get angry.

His adolescent rebellion consisted of informing his father he would not go to law school and spend his career arguing, but that he wanted to become a doctor.

He had no trouble in college, because he used the same philosophy he had learned earlier. Do what the teachers ask, and a good grade will be the reward. Harry was not a gifted science student, but he managed to make the necessary A's and B's. He enjoyed electives in history and philosophy the most.

In medical school, he found everyone as conforming as he, except many of his classmates were smarter and most were passionately interested in science. Virtually everyone studied hard, and all competed for class standing. Many of the courses seemed irrelevant to taking care of patients, but Harry trusted the wisdom of those who designed the curriculum. He was optimistic that if he did what was asked of him, he would learn what he needed to become a good doctor.

He graduated in the upper third of his medical school class, and secured an internal medicine residency at a solid university hospital. His willingness to work got him through the sleepless nights and holidays on call. He did feel inadequate and chagrined when senior physicians picked apart his examinations and use of laboratory tests. This undid some of his previous self-confidence, but he never thought to question whether their badgering was constructive or sadistic. Whatever it took to become a good doctor, he would put up with it.

Working one hundred hours a week as a resident, he had very little time for outside activities. He usually treated himself to short weekly sanity breaks outside the University Hospital, at least to see a movie, or go to a ball game. He met his future wife, Carol, at a football tailgate party. She worked as a nurse in the intensive care unit at St. Egregius, a community hospital five miles away from the University. They immediately struck a common bond, being of the same religion, and both coming from nearby cities. Further, as they got closer, they learned their parents had several friends in common. Harry felt that sharing the same culture he did, Carol would understand his dream of becoming a great doctor.

They married after dating for eighteen months, but they actually didn't know each other very well. Carol became morose whenever Harry had to work holidays. That got worse when they had a baby. For the first time in his life, Harry began to feel torn between conflicting desires and duties. He loved Carol and his new daughter, Katie, but he felt responsible not to leave his patients.

Harry refused to let these disturbing thoughts distract him from his goal, and he single-mindedly applied himself to become certified by the American Board. In addition, while at the University, he carried out a clinical research project treating cancer patients with tranquilizers to reduce their need for narcotics.

The more successful he was at the University, the less successful he was at home. It seemed like he was developing two parallel lives, and the people in one didn't understand the other. Carol began to refer to University Hospital as the concrete mistress. Every time he spent a few extra minutes in the clinic with a problem patient, he worried he was neglecting Katie.

Harry and Carol survived the training period, however, and both hoped it would be different in practice. Harry would have more control over his schedule. He also consoled himself with the notion that in return for his being willing to work at night, see sick people on weekends and holidays, and keep up on new medical advances, his material needs would be met. He repeated it over and over to himself; do a good job and people will reward you. Patients need your skills. Just worry about giving good care.

This worked, not wonderfully, but well enough. Harry's practice grew over the first five years. He and Carol did live in a nice house, plus had enough money for vacations and baby sitters. Harry even took up golf as he settled into the life of a practicing doctor.

He tried his best to cure his patients, to relieve their suffering, and prolong their lives. But as time went on, something just didn't seem to be working. He started to wonder whether it was all worth it. Despite his efforts, patients still kept getting sick. Those who were overweight stayed fat. The smokers developed heart and lung problems but continued to puff away. The alcoholics kept relapsing, and it was always on a weekend.

The hospital, once an exciting place to work, seemed to be a site of gloom. It was the last stop for the elderly who had no place to go and no one to care about them. Some had undergone high-risk operations that left them forever malnourished, infected, and depressed. So many of them were at the end, dying of chronic illnesses that had ravaged them for years. And no matter how hard he tried, Harry couldn't cure them.

And there were patients with advanced AIDS. Those poor suffering souls, wasted and demented, demanding and resentful. Enraged that they had been stricken by the disease, bitter at being isolated, angry at the pain.

It seemed like everyone was hostile. The patients and their families accused the doctors of being preoccupied and remote. They were irritated at the nurses who were so focused on their routines that they rarely took time to comfort the sick.

The hospital was noisy, cluttered, and chaotic. An array of reviewers was constantly checking to see what patients could be moved home, or out to a convalescent hospital. Filling out forms and documenting treatments took more and more of everyone's time. It was certainly not a place conducive to healing.

Harry felt like he was always rushed. No matter how hard he tried to meet his patients' needs, there was always more to do. He meant to be on time for his appointments in the office, but patients often had multiple complaints, or an emergency came up. When this happened the patients would become irate, and his office staff would be exasperated.

Some of his fellow doctors had grown cynical. They paid attention only to what was minimally necessary and called consultants to take care of other problems. They didn't want to bother talking to patients, particularly those with inconsequential worries. They drove nice cars, went on glamorous vacations, and seemed to have found a way to beat the system. But beneath the veneer of success, their complaining spread like a poisonous cloud from the doctors' dining room.

Harry knew he worked hard. Certainly his family knew it. Carol resented the time he spent on committees at the hospital. Yet he had to be sure the patients were getting good care. Sometimes Katie acted cross about sharing her dad with sick patients. He never thought it would turn out this way. He had envisioned himself in a white coat, curing patients, and receiving Christmas baskets from the most grateful ones.

Now, so much had changed. Many patients were grateful, and he did get gifts at Christmas. But many patients were hostile and expected him to be perfect. They wouldn't give him room to be impatient or make a mistake. They complained about his fees and challenged whether his services were even necessary. Many were leaving to join health plans, apologizing that they liked him but wanted to save money.

A few had even sent letters threatening to sue him. Thank goodness no one had actually gone through with it, but he knew many colleagues who had undergone the humiliating ordeal of anxiety, depositions, and court appearances.

Dealing with health plans was overwhelming him. He received obscure letters in legalese every week, piling on extra tasks or challenging his judgments. He became infuriated to read of the millions of dollars being amassed by insurance companies. He knew they were profiting from his efforts.

He found himself questioning whether he had made a mistake when he went to medical school. The training had been so long; eight years after college putting up with arrogant professors and uncooperative administrators. He had been thirty years old and heavily in debt when he started into practice.

He had put aside social contacts while he passed his certifying boards. He always seemed to be postponing his own desires for someone else's good. And now, at the peak of his career, he still had uneasy feelings that he wasn't doing enough.

One day in late winter, while he was in a really low mood, he even began to wonder if life itself was worth it. Did he really want to go on living this way? He was getting to the point where he couldn't enjoy anything. Sleep wasn't refreshing; food was tasteless. He realized that he wasn't just stale, he was depressed. He had fulminating burn-out, and had to act.

# Chapter 2.

# Seeking a Sage

**H**arry knew he needed help. What colleagues could he trust enough to talk about his distress? How about clergy? Harry didn't attend religious services regularly and he felt awkward about asking for counseling at his church. One night he got a telephone call from an older physician named Sanford Hayworth. Hayworth practiced in another part of the city and they knew each other casually. He recalled Harry's research at the University hospital. They had worked together on several committees of the county medical society. He wanted to know if Harry would serve on a task force to develop better pain treatment for cancer patients.

Harry had been impressed with Hayworth's affability and confidence. He wondered where they came from. He knew the senior man's practice couldn't be much different from his own. He must also have to cope with the frustrating changes. Hayworth always seemed to comment knowledgeably and wisely at meetings. Harry wondered how he managed not only to stay serene but to generate enthusiasm in others. Maybe it was because he had raised his children and no longer had heavy financial responsibilities. He probably had plenty salted away in his retirement plan. Easy for him to be happy. But Harry also knew Sanford Hayworth had been a mentor to medical society entrants, and helped physicians troubled by problems with alcohol or drugs. He had a reservoir of good will to give others. Maybe he could help.

Harry vacillated for three weeks, though he knew Hayworth was the one to call. Harry felt embarrassed to approach a colleague for advice, especially someone he didn't know intimately. Yet he knew he was depressed. Maybe someone he didn't know too well would be more objective. The days were getting longer, but winter wasn't giving way to spring without a fight. Harry's mood was as drab as the cold rains sweeping in from the west.

One drizzly day in March three patients cancelled office visits, which left his schedule light. He couldn't use being busy as an excuse to procrastinate. The sky was gray, and spray swirled under the eaves outside his consultation room. Harry felt distracted as he worked through his patients, planning what he would say to Sanford Hayworth. When 5 p.m. came, he knew he had to act if he was going to make any changes in his life. He took a deep breath and picked up the telephone. His fingers were clumsy as he hit the touch pads because he didn't know exactly what to say, and he didn't want a senior doctor to suspect he was an alcoholic or a drug abuser.

Sanford Hayworth came on the line, and Harry relaxed at the confident, reassuring manner he heard over the telephone. Harry described how he had observed his older colleague counsel new doctors. He said he knew of Hayworth's work with physicians impaired by depression. Harry struggled as he tried to put into words how exhausted he felt. Finally, he asked if there was any way they could talk in person, to get a consultation about his career in medicine.

"By all means," said Hayworth, "You know, I get a surprising number of calls from doctors who want to talk about their careers. There's a lot of concern about the future, a lot of disillusionment out there nowadays. I think I understand what you're feeling. Sounds like you need time out for healing. I'd be happy to meet and talk with you about it. What if we have breakfast together next week?"

"That would be great," said Harry, and he reached for his calendar. "How about next Tuesday morning? Is 7:30 okay for you?"

"Let's see, I don't start seeing patients in the office until 9:00 that day, so that should be fine."

They named a coffee shop half way between their offices. "Very good," said Harry. "I'll look forward to it."

He exhaled as he hung up the telephone. He put his fingers over his chin and began to muse. What did Sanford Hayworth mean by saying that he needed time out for healing? Did he mean healing himself, or healing others? Harry hoped Hayworth didn't think he was incompetent. He drove home that evening in the rain, slowly, and pensively.

That night he dreamed he saw Sanford Hayworth in a large auditorium, sitting behind a wooden table on the stage. Doctors were lined up to speak to him. There was a microphone on the table, and the audience, all white-coated physicians, were taking notes. When Harry got to the table, the dream ended, and he woke up.

Over the next few days, as he made his rounds and saw his office patients, Harry pondered that puzzling phrase, *time out for healing*. But he looked forward to the breakfast meeting. He had a hunch Sanford Hayworth would be able to help him.

When Tuesday arrived, he arose before sunrise. He exercised, and dressed carefully so that he would appear positive. It was overcast but mild, common weather for that time of year. An early morning shower had made the pavement shiny and Harry saw pencils of light breaking through the clouds as he drove to the meeting.

Sanford Hayworth was seated in a booth at one side of the restaurant scanning the menu. Harry headed toward him and both men shook hands. Hayworth was medium height and stocky. His hair was sandy gray, the crown thinning. His skin was ruddy and lined, like someone who works outdoors. He had thick gray eyebrows arching over inquisitive eyes that danced when they looked at Harry.

Both ordered from the so-called "low fat" menu. They laughed as they compared cholesterol levels. After the coffee had been poured, Sanford Hayworth opened the conversation.

"Tell me then, what's been on your mind that made you telephone me? I took it as a compliment. As I get more gray hair, I'm getting more calls like yours."

Harry took a sip of coffee. "Well, it just seems like I'm getting stale. I've been in practice six years, and by most people's measure, I'm successful. Yet, there are times when I feel like a child trying to empty the ocean into a sand bucket."

"Are you disappointed? It's common for doctors five or six years into practice to realize that they can't cure most of their patients."

Harry picked up a teaspoon, and began to trace a circle on the paper mat at his place. "That's certainly part of it. It's just I work so hard, and my patients aren't improving."

"I remember when I went through that phase," the older man mused, looking over Harry's shoulder out the window. "I was just about your age. I'd been taught to diagnose complicated diseases, and to prescribe intricate treatments. I found that I was rushing more and enjoying practice less. I finally realized that I needed time out to think about healing."

Harry raised his eyebrows, perplexity on his face. "Tell me what you mean by 'think about healing'? Of course I think about healing. I want to heal all my patients. Healing is my vocation. Curing diseases is how I do it."

"That's my point. The measure of success isn't curing. Most of the time, we don't do much curing at all. You remember the quote from Ambrose Pare, the French surgeon four hundred years ago. 'I dressed the wound and God healed it'? When a cure occurs, it's usually because of something the patient does. Any doctor who focuses on curing and measures his or her success on cure rates is going to be frustrated. Healing and curing aren't the same thing by any means."

Harry stopped making loops with the teaspoon. "Okay. Are you saying I should quit worrying about curing my patients, and emphasize healing as a different goal?"

"To some extent. Another quote: 'To cure occasionally, to treat sometimes, to comfort always.' Remember that one?"

Harry chuckled, and tilted his chin upward knowingly. "I remember being told that in medical school. But you know, I don't think many of us pay much attention to it under the tremendous pressure to treat. Patients and colleagues demand results."

Hayworth took a sip of his coffee before continuing. "Absolutely. That's a major obstacle to healing, the rush that results from the pressure to treat. Particularly here in the U. S., we're activists. We're a nation of doers. We pride ourselves on going out and solving problems. We're like mechanics, looking for things to fix. Sometimes we need to be more like gardeners, and let nature heal."

He wiped his lips with his napkin. "We all make mistakes occasionally. You know if you make a mistake that it'll be much easier to defend something you did wrong, rather than something you neglected to do."

Harry thought back to his days in training. How many times had he been pilloried for overlooking some test or procedure? But not if he tried something that failed. He had come to take it for granted that patients want something done. "Why would a patient come to the doctor if he doesn't want to be treated?" he asked defensively.

"People come for many reasons; reassurance, comfort, peace of mind. Sometimes just to be around other humans. It's a failing of our culture that we insist on pills or operations as signs of a cure. I admit, our patients fall into the same traps we doctors do, and so I don't want to pick on you. My point is people respond to symbols. Deep down they seek to be healed. The symbols may not have anything to do with curing, because often, curing isn't possible."

Hayworth's voice slowed and he looked deep into Harry's eyes. "Healing is almost always possible, however. If you want to continue to be a healer, and I'm sure you do, I can help you."

Harry was skeptical. He had been to seminars on healing and holistic medicine. The speakers always seemed to have ponytails and wear flannel shirts. They typically had no formal medical training after internship. He had dismissed them as unscientific weirdoes.

The waitress approached their booth with two steaming glass coffee pots. "Would you gentlemen like refills?" she asked, extending the orange collared decaffeinated sphere toward them.

"Enough for me," said Hayworth, putting his palm over his cup. As she retreated, he looked over and chided Harry. "Be tolerant. Yes, there are some phonies out there promoting touchy-feely medicine, but we in the mainstream sometimes get so arrogant about our roots in science, that we close our minds. People are a lot more than a collection of interacting organs.

"They're starting to see this in the medical schools. Over at the University there's a course being offered called Values in Medicine. Even the professors are coming to see its benefit, and most of them have made their careers concentrating on some narrow area of research."

Harry's eyes brightened. He hadn't thought a lot about the distinction between healing and curing, but he did know about the Values in Medicine course. The more he considered it, the more it made sense. Curing relates to getting rid of diseases and focuses on pathology. Healing relates to recovery, to restoring wholeness, and to the person. Healing depends on doctor and patient recognizing and respecting each other's values.

"All right," he said with a trace of humility, "I see what you mean. What's the trick to becoming a healer?"

"You already are a healer," laughed Hayworth. "You just need some of the steam wiped off your mirror so that you can see yourself better.

"In fact, I'd say you're a gifted healer. I've worked with you. You're considerate and compassionate. I think your problems relate to being obsessively compassionate." Hayworth motioned to the waitress for the check.

Harry was confused. Being obsessively compassionate sounded like a description of exactly the kind of physician he wanted to be. He felt annoyed. "Being thorough is the mark of a good doctor."

The older man responded. "You're even compulsive now as you think about what I'm saying. The important distinction is how much. You're getting the doctor's disease; you're developing into an excessive obsessive-compulsive.

"Look, there are a lot of changes occurring in medicine now. Doctors try to manage change by staying in control, but that's getting tougher and tougher. You can't do it, and I can't do it."

Hayworth looked at his wristwatch. "Well, it's getting late now. We both have to get to our rounds. Let's plan to have another meeting next week. In the meantime, think about it. A little bit of compulsivity makes us do a good job. Too much makes us frustrated when we can't control our environment."

Harry was still confused. But, he agreed to meet again. He thanked his colleague, and left the coffee shop. The sun was up, but the water had not fully evaporated from the pavement. Silver puddles glistened along the streets as he drove to the hospital. He found himself more perplexed than before.

Where was the line between thoroughness and obsessiveness? Was he a control freak? He wasn't sure. Through his mind percolated Sanford Hayworth's diagnosis: an excessive focus on curing. The treatment? Time out for healing.

# Chapter 3.

# Socrates with a Scissors

After seeing his patients at the hospital the next morning, Harry decided he needed a haircut. He walked down the street to Mel's barber shop, where he had been a customer ever since he started in practice. He walked in, waved at Mel, and sat down to read the sports page of the morning newspaper while he waited his turn.

Melchior Filipone was five feet seven, and had to stand on a stool to reach the heads of his tallest customers. He had a fringe of black hair around the back of his head, but the top was shiny bald. He had to endure jokes that he rarely needed his own services. His skin was olive, and he shaved twice daily because his beard grew so thick within six hours it made him look sinister. His fingers were short and stubby, but they became a blur of motion when he went to work with his scissors. Mel greeted Harry with a ritual question, "So what's up, Doc?"

"Hell, Mel, I'm swell," replied Harry, reciting the ritual response, as he settled into a cracked red vinyl stuffed chair. He began to flip pages, scanning rather than reading the newspaper. In a few minutes, Mel motioned him to the chair, snapping a striped cloth sheet to get rid of a clump of hair left on the seat by the last patron.

Mel put a paper collar around Harry's neck, and fixed the drape tightly with a clip. "You don't look so hot, Doc. Something the matter?"

"I've been a little overworked lately. Sometimes it's tough to please everyone."

"For sure," commented Mel, nodding wisely. "Same thing here at the shop. One guy wants more off the top, the next wants the top left longer. Sometimes I wish I was back in the Army, where we just turned on the clippers and scalped 'em. We didn't have to take any lip from recruits. It always grows back in a month, anyhow."

"I've been feeling frustrated trying to figure out how to help my patients. No matter what I do, their diseases seem to have minds of their own."

"So, what d'you expect?" replied Mel. "They're sick, Doc. That's why they're coming to you. People who are well don't go to the doctor. When people are sick, they're not at their best."

"They're certainly not," responded Harry, shaking his head.

"Hold still, Doc. I don't want to snip your ear. Look. You make good money. You probably help a lot of the people who come to you. You have respect. I'd bet a bunch of guys within hailing distance of this shop would trade places with you."

"I know. I'm actually pretty lucky, for many of the reasons you just mentioned. Sometimes I get introspective."

Harry blushed. He had been reluctant to talk to a fellow doctor about his feelings and here he was getting into psychological analysis with his barber. "What drives you?" asked Mel. "I don't think it's money. I've been cutting your hair long enough to know that. I think you're an idealist, and the fate of idealists is to be disappointed."

Mel stopped cutting Harry's sideburns, and pointed the scissors at him. "It's like barbering. I trim people's hair, and it makes them look nice. Some people have funny shaped heads, and I can actually disguise the bumps. Some people are vain, and if I please them, they give me a fat tip. Sometimes they're dissatisfied, and they don't give me any tip.

"But you know what? When the hair's been cut, it gets swept into the trash, and in a month, it grows back. That's just the way things are. Nature is out to undo what I do as a barber."

"I never thought of barbers as frustrating Nature," laughed Harry.

"I don't frustrate Nature, I enhance her," retorted Mel indignantly. "But the hair grows back. No matter how artistic I am today, you're head is going to be shaggy in six weeks and you'll have to come back.

He looked out the window onto the street at a bus passing by. "All of us, you, me, the guy driving that bus, we do our job, put a little sunshine in another person's life, and then enjoy ourselves after work.

"Doc, I got to tell you, I see some gray hairs here. You're thinking too hard. Keep it simple. You know what I'm thinking about right now? Tonight for dinner Sophie's going to make osso bucco. It's my favorite. A little pasta, vino, that's what I'm looking forward to. Tomorrow there'll be another twenty people in this shop to get clipped."

"Mel, that's why I come to this shop. I not only get a hair cut, I get counseling."

Mel resumed his trimming, lifting tufts of Harry's hair with a comb, and snipping deftly. "I've got a customer. Rich guy. Owns a construction company. Crusty old geezer. Hard to please. One time he was in here getting his hair cut when someone from his office called, and it must have bugged him. He gave the guy hell over the phone, ranting at him with all the other customers listening.

"He got back in this chair, right where you are now, and he says to me, 'Mel, you know why all of us exist?' I say to him I don't know, and he says to me, 'we're all here to make things a little bit easier for others.'

"Doc, that was profound. And you know, the guy was right. Why make it more complicated than that?

"Sometimes I think you doctors and lawyers have IQ's that are too high for your own good. Life's to be lived, not analyzed."

"Mel, you're a tonsorial Plato."

"Hey, the Socrates of the scissors, that's me," boasted Mel. "So, who d'you think'll pitch on opening day for the Yankees?"

"Pettitte," said Harry.

"Unless they go with Clemens or Cone," countered Mel. And with that change of subject, the two of them proceeded to discuss whether New York would have any chance to repeat as world's champs.

After carefully combing Harry's hair, Mel pulled off the sheet, and sent him on his way. "Remember, Doc, just make life a little easier for the other guy. Don't complicate it more than that. Too much thinking causes gray hair. See you in a month."

Harry was laughing as he pulled shut the door to the shop. He walked back to the hospital replaying Mel's philosophy in his own mind: make life easier for others, and don't overanalyze.

## Chapter 4.

# Time Out for Healing

**T**he following Tuesday morning Harry felt exhilarated. Spring was definitely coming. A cloudless sky let the rising sun turn the hills east of the city various shades of green and yellow. Pine trees in his back yard shone light green at their tops, dark green at their bases, and gray blue where their shadows fell over the dewy grass. Harry contrasted his own mood with the previous week. This time he wasn't apprehensive; he was eager.

The sun that had turned the trees in Harry's yard green was brightening the washed walls of the still quiet coffee shop when he pulled open the glass entry door. At the counter two patrons in jeans and boots, probably carpenters or electricians on their way to work, were chuckling over some shared joke amidst scrambled eggs and toast. Sanford Hayworth was at the same booth in the corner where he had been last week. Harry slid onto the seat across from him. Again they shook hands. "This is one of those mornings I love to get up," said Hayworth. "Last night I had a meeting about the wellness program for the elderly the mayor has been pushing, and I didn't get a chance to see the sun go down. The days are just long enough for it to be light when I finish at the office and I hate to miss the sunset. We have enough cloudy afternoons at this time of the year, that I need those sunsets. They make evening come peacefully. I felt a little deprived last night."

They placed their breakfast orders, and Hayworth spoke again. "Last week, we started to talk about control, and its relation to healing, wasn't that it?"

"Something like that," responded Harry. "You were urging me to be a little bit compulsive, but no more."

"Rigid habits are a defense against worry. It's natural to feel uncertain about the future. There's no way any of us could have been expected to foresee the social changes occurring today. We're victims of 'future shock'. That's not just a cliché. It isn't just us. Our patients are having a tough time. I know you're frustrated, but I'll bet your patients are as well."

"They're nearly as bewildered as I am," said Harry. "They feel bounced around by insurance companies. The claims forms alone are sadistically complex. They must be designed to confuse patients. People don't like to be treated like a set of numbers. They do wish it were simpler, like the old days. They don't like the forms, but their pocketbooks are protected by the very maze they resent."

"Definitely. Megacorporations in medicine are intimidating. There's real danger that both patients and doctors will be turned into commodities, look alike products that are only told apart from one another by their price."

Hayworth sighed, as he looked out the window for a moment at the passing traffic. "There was a time when I was confused and dispirited. I've learned there's a better way to live." He turned back, and looked at Harry. "Whenever physicians like you come to me with stories like yours, I tell them about that better way. I call it 'time out for healing.'"

"You used that term last week. What exactly do you mean? I wasn't sure if the term healing referred to me healing my patients, or me being healed."

Hayworth smiled. "Healing refers to healing yourself. You know the old adage about the wounded healer. Well, we all have some head wounds. But if we can just get the right perspective, we do a better job, and we enjoy our lives more.

"When I talk about time out for healing, I mean standing aside and taking stock. It's a process. It involves several steps. In fact, there are several mentors who can help you, right here in our city. Some of them helped me, and I've helped some of them. I'll introduce you to them."

He paused again to put jelly on a piece of whole-wheat toast. "Some of them are doctors just like you and me. Some are nurses. We M. D.'s have a lot to learn from the R. N.'s. Some are ex-patients, if there is such a thing. Let's start with the art of listening. I think the first person you should talk with is Leslie Ladd. She's a world class listener. Give her a call. I'll let her know you'll be phoning her. Does that sound okay?"

Harry shifted in the booth, and stretched his arm over the seat back. "If you say so. But that's part of my burnout. I'm exhausted listening, and I don't really want to talk with other people right now." he said. "It took just about all my energy to talk to you. I'm not up to blabbering my innermost thoughts to other doctors. I didn't sign up for group therapy."

"Talk to Leslie. You'll get a new perspective on listening, and this isn't group therapy, but it is insightful," chuckled Hayworth. "That's what living is about, making life a little easier for others."

Harry wondered where Sanford Hayworth got his hair cut.

Hayworth scrutinized his watch. "I'd like to talk more, but I have to supervise a treadmill test at Community Clinic, and I don't want to be late. After you speak with Leslie, give me a phone call. I'll be interested in your reaction." He rose, and whisked the check into his hand. "This breakfast's on me."

"I guess morning sun brings out generosity." remarked Harry.

"It's the promise of a spring day that does it," smiled Sanford Hayworth. "And the pleasure of sending a new friend on an adventure." He waved to Harry, pulled his car keys from his pocket, and unlocked the door of his dark blue Buick sedan.

Harry stood in front of the coffee shop for a minute as he watched the older man back out of the parking slot. Hayworth put on sunglasses, pulled down the windshield visor, and waved again to Harry as he swung into the street.

Harry drove to his office from the coffee shop analyzing Hayworth's theme. Stand aside. Call time out for healing.

## Chapter 5.

# *Medical Music*

That evening Harry went home elated. The trees in his front yard were charcoal colored in the fading light of the early spring sunset. Wispy gray and orange clouds blended with the silhouettes of the hills to the west. Porch lights were on throughout his neighborhood. He clicked the garage door opener, a luxury Carol insisted he have to neutralize the discomfort of midnight trips to the hospital. He turned off the car lights, and entered the kitchen. He smelled basil and thyme in a casserole simmering in the oven.

He walked in and looked at Carol. She was dressed in a red ribbed turtleneck sweater and jeans that showed off her figure. Carol was nearly as tall as Harry, and thin, with straight black hair that she usually pulled back in a ponytail. She had dark eyes, high cheekbones, and a softly curved chin. Her face was too long to be characterized as truly beautiful, but she was a very nice looking woman, particularly as far as Harry was concerned. She wore little makeup, which Harry felt reinforced her natural attractiveness.

He kissed her, put his arm around her waist, and held her for several seconds, which seemed to disconcert her. He picked up Katie to swirl her around the kitchen. Carol was surprised, and said, "What got into you? It's not payday. Harry, what's going on?"

"Just say that I had an insightful experience today."

"Can you tell me?" Carol inquired, donning quilted mittens to open the lid of the casserole.

"Sure, I had breakfast this morning with Sanford Hayworth. You know him, don't you? He's the chair of the New Physician Committee at the County Medical Society. Believe it or not, we talked about taking time out for healing."

Harry then proceeded to relate his conversation with Dr. Hayworth. Carol nodded as she listened. She went to the refrigerator and pulled out a bottle of salad dressing. She poured it over a bowl of shredded lettuce, turning the leaves with a large spoon. Finally she spoke up. "Harry, you're really hard on yourself. I often wish there were something I could do to get you to let up. You have such high standards in everything you do. The rest of us mortals find it difficult to keep up with you."

Harry sat down, put Katie on his lap and hugged her, rocking slowly. "I'm trying to learn, Carol," he said.

Considering how good he felt all day, Harry slept poorly that night. He dreamed he was pushing a string across a table. Sanford Hayworth was behind him, urging him on. Carol was holding the far end of the string. Every time he pushed, the string buckled. He kept telling Hayworth, "I can't do this. The string keeps buckling. I can't get the force straight."

Hayworth moved to Carol's end of the string, and gently pulled it straight. "Try it from this end," he suggested. "Pulling will be easier."

"No, no, I have to push it," Harry kept objecting. But the string kept bending, and looping. Harry's frustration mounted, and he finally woke up.

The next morning Harry drove silently through rush hour traffic. He wanted to think. He was perplexed. Leslie Ladd was a dermatologist. He didn't know her well, but he had met her. She seemed articulate, that much he had observed, but how could a dermatologist be a world class listener? Dermatologists look at spots and lesions. They're not listeners.

He thought he didn't have much to lose by talking with her, and so Harry called her office at noon that day. She came on the other end of the line, and when he said he was calling at the suggestion of Sanford Hayworth, she replied she would be happy to meet him.

"He and I have been friends for years," said Leslie Ladd. "We've spent many good times together talking about what it means to be a competent physician. He helped me develop a talk on medical music that I present at dermatology meetings. Let's get together and I'll summarize it for you. I start my office early to accommodate patients that have to go to work, but next Thursday I could start later if that would be convenient for you."

"Thursday, 7 a.m. looks fine to me," Harry answered. "Name the place." They arranged to meet at her office.

The week was busy for Harry. He had two consultations at the hospital every day, and was managing three patients in the critical care unit. Added were the inevitable calls at night from the nurses, reporting laboratory tests, and seeking reassurance about changes in vital signs. Despite these distractions, he kept musing to himself. "The listening dermatologist, medical music; this is incongruous."

Thursday morning at 7 a.m. he was waiting at her door when Dr. Leslie Ladd arrived. She was a small woman.

Harry guessed her to be five feet two, and between forty-five and fifty years old. She was trim however, and she carried herself with the stride of fitness. Her hair was gray-brown and curly. Her features were smooth and symmetrical. She wore stylish glasses, and a scarf around her neck.

She moved fast, and came right up to him. They shook hands, and she invited him in. She opened louvered shutters in the reception room, and seated Harry in a consultation room that seemed appropriate for her size. She stepped into an alcove where she began to boil water, and fetched tea bags out of a cupboard above. "I like a cup of hot tea on these chilly spring mornings," she commented, then called to Harry, "Would you like me to make you tea or instant coffee?"

"I'd like coffee," he called back. Harry looked about the room. It was small, and manifested femininity, with pastel upholstery on the chairs, and a fruitwood desk standing on curved legs. Pictures of a young woman in a cap and gown and a middle-aged man were displayed on a credenza beneath the usual diplomas and certificates. Presumably her husband and daughter.

A large window behind the desk gave a westward view of the inner courtyard of the office building. Harry figured she sought afternoon sun to work without artificial light most of the time.

Leslie Ladd made a few opening inquiries about his practice that Harry recognized as icebreakers since they knew each other only slightly. Then gently, even casually, she said, "Tell me what prompted your call last week." Though a sparkle remained in her eye and she was smiling, Harry could feel her antennae going up, like from a car whose driver has just turned on the radio.

He recapped for her the frustrations he was feeling in his practice, how the patients were so demanding, how third party payers and government agencies seemed almost to delight in complicating life, and how the rewards he sought just didn't seem to be there any more.

She didn't speak. She just nodded a few times as though she was trying to encourage him. After he stopped, it seemed like she consciously paused before responding. "The rewards are there," she said. "But, I agree, it's often difficult to perceive them. Can you specify any things that do give you pleasure in your practice?"

"Sure. I have a lot of nice people as my patients. They're interesting. They've done a lot of worthwhile things with their lives. Some of them are admirable. There are some jerks, too, of course, but they're the minority.

"Because I've been in practice a while, and because of my research, I get quite a few referrals for consultation. When I have to arouse the old cerebral cortex, concentrate and use my skills, that gets the adrenaline going, and I like it. It doesn't seem like there are so many of those any more."

"Why do you suppose that is?" she replied. "You're known for being expert. I would expect your referral rate to be climbing."

Harry was forced to concede. He re-crossed his legs, and self-consciously tickled his ear lobe. "Actually, I track this in the office, and you're right. My referral rates are pretty steady. It's that they don't seem as preponderant as they once were."

"So, it's not the composition of your practice that's changed, but how you see it," she commented.

"You may be right, looking at it that way."

"I'm sure you're just as good as you were ten years ago," she went on. "In fact, you're probably better because your base of experience is broader and deeper now. I'd expect that would please you. The patients are the same, their illnesses are the same, and your skill is better. That ought to be a formula for contentment."

"If you simplify it to that point, it sounds like the practice is going well," he agreed.

"That's the key," she said. "We have to simplify things. That's why listening is so important, for you to help your patients, or for me to help you.

"Doctors sometimes act like they have to have sophisticated answers to all questions to help patients. That's not really the way it is. We help them by hearing them out. That's how it works, and why it works."

Harry could see that she was warming up. She leaned forward over the desk top, and folded her hands with the index fingers pointing upward. "People keep trying to understand exactly what it is that doctors do that helps heal. Part of the answer is being present. Presence and listening are part of the healing. I don't mean silence. Silence doesn't convey any message. I mean listening, an active engagement with the patient.

"That's why when I'm talking about this I use the term medical music. Medical music is the harmony that results from the doctor listening and resonating back to the patient. Something very mysterious occurs, very primitive, and very much part of the human spirit. Like music, it's universal." She stopped to let him absorb what she said.

Harry didn't reply, and so she went on, speaking faster. "The same process applies in dealing with colleagues.

Have you ever been presenting a case, and been interrupted? You want to say, 'Stop a second and let me explain why I want your help.' Doctors are like many others. They're bright enough that they pick up on parts of what people say, fill in the blanks, and think they heard the message. Often they haven't. And unfortunately that not only prevents healing from taking place, it can lead to mistakes, and harm to patients. With lawsuits for dessert. This becomes doubly important if the patient is new, or unknown. It's true even for dermatologists, who may see patients only for short periods of time for very specific problems."

"I know what you mean, but I don't think I've ever quite thought of it that way." said Harry. "Listening takes only a tiny extra amount of time up front, but it saves lots of time later and makes medicine work better. That's what you're saying."

She nodded. "Listening isn't the whole thing, and I don't want to shortchange the other faculties that promote healing. But it's the keystone. That's true for teachers, architects, sales people, and even parents." She pointed toward the picture of her daughter to the side.

"If you're interested in going into this further, I can suggest another very helpful person for you to call."

"Who's that?"

"Do you know Len Spector, the pathologist?" she asked.

"Just by reputation," said Harry. "He runs the lab at St. Paradox, doesn't he?"

"Yes. And he's an expert on internal limits. You should consider talking to him."

"Thanks. But what do you mean by internal limits? When I say "limits" to patients or their families, it connotes failure to reach the goal. I tell someone with cancer, 'Yes Mrs. Jones, there are limits to what we can do. I'm sorry. But I can't do more.'"

"Go talk to Len." she said. "He'll explain what he means by limits. Considering he works on dead cells and reagents all day, he's a really insightful person."

"All right," said Harry. "I promise I'll give him a call."

He rose and shook her hand. Her mannerisms reminded Harry of one of his high school teachers who would come out from behind her desk to say good bye to the students as they filed out of the classroom. He thought for a second. Leslie Ladd was senior enough to have been his teacher.

As he drove to his office, Harry thought more about what she said. Listening to patients helps simplify healing. Medical music is the harmony between the doctor and the patient when the patient feels heard.

*Chapter 6.*

# *Internal Limits*

The next day, Harry called the St. Paradox laboratory.

"Dr. Len Spector? Leslie Ladd referred me to you. She and I had a great session yesterday on the art of listening, and she said I should talk to you. She used the term 'internal limits' and said you are the limit expert."

On the other end of the telephone line, Harry could hear him chuckle. "Yes, Leslie's a fine lady. The only dermatologist I know who uses her ears as much as her eyes and fingers. She and I have become friends over the years, and when we start to get serious, talking about the meaning of life and such, I always remind her of how I had to learn to be imperfect."

"That seems like a strange way to put it," said Harry. "None of us has to learn to be imperfect; we're born that way."

"Right. But for us M. D.'s, the system tries to turn us into perfectionists. That's why we get tied in knots. If you want to come over to St. Par's and meet me, I'll tell you the story of my self-awareness safari. It'll explain what I mean."

The following day, after he had finished his morning rounds, Harry called to be sure Dr. Spector was available. He then drove over to St. Paradox Hospital, and went to the pathology department.

He found the little office of Dr. Spector amidst the centrifuges and multi-channel analyzers. Seated behind the side return of a low, flat desk, squinting through a micro-scope, was the senior pathologist.

Spector was short, bald, and wore thick glasses. He reminded Harry of a film critic on one of the television networks.

"Glad to see you," said Spector. "Do you have a little time? Let me finish dictating this surgical, and I'll be right with you." He flipped a foot switch and proceeded to describe the findings on the slide. In a minute, he stopped, switched off the microscope light, and put the slide in a cardboard holder. He swung around in his chair to face Harry, and started to talk.

"When I was in medical school and was an intern, I got the idea that one can never be too careful. There's always another test that can be done. The patient can always be checked again. Maybe we missed something the first time around.

"Go back to your own internship. Remember a morning after a night on call? You had no sleep, and you admitted four sick patients. One died after you spent three hours trying to get her out of shock.

"Now, it's 9 a.m., and the chief resident, or even better, the senior attending physician, comes onto the floor for rounds. You feel terrible. Your saliva's dry and your con-junctival capillaries look like roads of red ink. Your hair is tousled, and you have twenty-four hours of stubble on your chin.

"Have you ever had an attending look at you and say, 'You must have been up all night. Go to bed and get some rest.'? No, more likely he asked why you didn't have the latest hemoglobin level on the patient in room six ten, or if you checked the results of the morning blood sugars on your diabetic patients.

"My point is, you can never do enough. There's always more, no matter how thorough and diligent you may be."

Spector pushed his glasses upward on his round nose and went on. "We were taught it was a sign of weakness to delegate responsibilities. To rely on the judgment of a nurse or laboratory technician was a sign of character weakness. 'No competent doctor asks another person to do a task he can't do himself.' Ever heard that?"

Harry smiled wistfully. "I sure have. I remember in my senior year in medical school, we had a resident who had to take down every bit of the history and record it long-hand. His histories were ten pages long. And he printed them. He ordered every test the lab could perform. The senior staff loved him, but the rest of us hated working with him, because he could only take care of one patient in an evening. We had to work up most of his admissions."

"No doubt," replied Len Spector. "And I'll bet you had a staff endocrinologist who could always think of some bio-chemical test you didn't order on a consultation. The system cultivates, and in a perverse way, rewards these eccentrics."

"The reason I went into pathology was in order to master the ultimate answer. I wanted to be able to know the last word. I nearly went crazy before I woke up."

"What do you mean?" asked Harry.

Spector began to gesture. Harry could see he how strongly he felt about what he was saying. "I was obsessed. I couldn't ever do a good enough job, and I blamed myself if things went wrong."

"Finally, I had a scary experience that made me think. I was in charge of the chemistry section. The lab accidentally reported out the serum potassium as 2.5, when it was really 5.2, in a patient with kidney insufficiency. The doctors in charge of the patient began to give the patient extra potassium, and he developed an irregular cardiac rhythm. Fortunately, he got over it, but when they repeated the test, and saw the mistake, I was devastated. I felt like it was my fault. I had nothing to do with it, but I felt responsible, and guilty.

"My chief took me aside, and played psychiatrist to me. He told me about human fallibility and the burden I was taking on if I insisted on perfection."

Spector stopped momentarily. His voice slowed down and he intoned, "He introduced me to the difference between excellence and perfection. Doing the best you can with what you have, in contrast to performing a task without an error or mistake. Of course, humans are inherently imperfect. But that doesn't mean we don't shoot for perfection. And when we do that as we care for patients, we really turn them into objects. We're not so much caring for another human as trying to show our ability to carry out a task perfectly."

The office was dead silent as Spector waited to see how Harry took what he said. Harry looked at the little pathologist, and at the microscope between them. It was the symbol of the deep search for medical facts.

Harry nodded assent. Cardboard trays of slides were stacked on both sides of Dr. Spector's desk. On the slides fixed in plastic were thin sheets of actual cells that had been alive not long ago, dividing and growing. Now they were just complex molecules stained purple and orange. It seemed out of place. Spector the pathologist, was a philosopher and a psychologist as well.

Spector resumed talking. "After that I began to share some of my thoughts and self doubts with my fellow residents and junior staff. At first, I was a little afraid because I wanted to maintain that aura of confidence. But the fact that my own chief, senior and wiser, had brought up the subject, freed me to reveal these thoughts to my fellow pathology residents.

"And an amazing thing happened. The more I shared of my ambivalence, the more the other residents helped me. It turned out they were having a lot of the same anxiety about how to be as perfect as the profession seemed to demand. It was great, because I got more support from them than I had ever experienced. They were more willing to help me with tough diagnoses and would give me opinions on surgicals. They really knew me. We really felt like we were on the same team. And it was all because I had simply opened up a bit to them."

Just then Spector's telephone rang, and he reached over to the receiver. He punched a button and greeted an anonymous caller. Harry listened as the pathologist's head bobbed up and down across from him. Then Spector asked the caller if they could continue the conversation later. He cradled the receiver, and looked back at Harry.

He said, "Physicians are complex. They usually aren't terribly introspective, in the sense that they don't think much about how what they do fits in the big picture. Or if they do, they exaggerate their own importance. On the other hand, they absorb guilt easily. They have a lot of self-doubt. That's good for patients, when it means they question a tentative diagnosis, or double-check what they are doing. It's bad for the doctors as human beings, because it leads them to strive compulsively to do things just right, and that gets other parts of life out of balance. A psychiatrist named Glen Gabbard has written a lot about this. Look up his work."

"Pretty deep stuff," commented Harry. "And not too pleasant for us M.D.'s to hear about ourselves."

"Getting doctors to engage in self-examination can be a struggle," said Spector. "That's what I meant by them being a complex species. It's that paradox; compulsive and obsessive about perfection and detail in what they do, but lacking introspection."

"How did you retrain yourself out of those tendencies?" asked Harry.

Spector intertwined his hands behind his head, as though he had expected that question. He leaned back lazily and Harry recognized pleasure in his voice. "Well, once I learned to accept an occasional mistake as the price of being a human being, and how to grow beyond the self recrimination that follows a mistake, it simply became a matter of setting up systems beforehand to minimize mistakes, and then taking things as they come."

"It's all a matter of how much of a control freak you have to be," said Dr. Spector. "It relates to being able to lead and guide without dominating and stifling."

"Sure," said Harry. "It's just like being a parent. One has to lead and guide children, but let them grow, and accept that they'll make mistakes."

"Sometimes with children, you do have to control and dominate them," said Len Spector. "But I think you get the overall sense of what I'm saying. Giving up total control in return for the chance to lead and influence. That's the message.

"On that note, I should really get you to call Charlie Sharp. He's the guru on control of control. Do you know him?"

"Sure, everyone knows Charles Sharp," replied Harry. "He's Chief of Surgery over at Summit General. Used to be a professor up at the University. He's invented surgical techniques and operations for conditions that previously couldn't even be approached. Very creative person."

"Definitely. But what you probably don't know is how he modulates his compulsions to control. He doesn't write much about it, but he does impart it to his residents. He's willing to share his thoughts with anyone who takes the trouble to ask him. Why don't you give him a call? Let him know you and I have been stamping out perfectionism. That'll do for an introduction."

"Len, thanks for all your help," said Harry, rising from his chair. "I'll be sure to get in touch with Dr. Sharp."

He left the lab, thinking as he passed the bright trays of stains and smelled the fixatives, that he never expected to learn psychology from a pathologist. He laughed at himself for being closed minded. Got to keep the old thinker open to new ideas, he thought as he drove back to his office from St. Paradox pathology lab. The message kept popping up in his mind: Excellently imperfect means doing the best with what we have

## Chapter 7.

# Control of Control

That evening Harry was again in high spirits as he drove home and greeted Carol and Katie. "You'll never guess where I went today," he said.

When he got no immediate reply he continued. "I visited with Len Spector, a pathologist at St. Paradox. We talked about being imperfect. I know it sounds crazy. Sanford Hayworth really gets the credit. He's the one who started me a few weeks ago. Do you remember when we went to breakfast that day? I've been on a quest since then, and I'm starting to see things more clearly than ever before."

"Go wash your hands," Carol said both to Katie and Harry. She then turned to Harry and looked at him querulously. "Harry, I can't follow a thing you're saying. But your mood's better. I don't know why. Whatever it is you're doing, keep it up." With that comment, she walked around the kitchen counter and kissed his cheek. "Let's eat. You can tell me more later."

Harry savored chicken piccata and pasta. He even uncorked a bottle of white wine to add festivity to the occasion, which made Carol roll her eyes in disbelief. After dinner, he read to Katie, and while Carol put her to bed, he called Dr. Charles Sharp.

He knew of Sharp by reputation, as a senior staff surgeon at Summit General, and a member of several committees in the local medical society. He knew almost nothing about him personally. Harry proceeded to relate what Len Spector had said.

Sharp listened quietly, not interrupting. Then he responded. "Control, control, the doctor's nemesis. I fought that demon for years before I came to understand how it was controlling me. If you're sincere about getting some insights on control, I'd be happy to help you. Let's meet, and I can share my thoughts. I usually operate on Monday, Wednesday, and Friday, but we could meet on Thursday here at Summit if you want."

"Thursday would work for me," said Harry, glancing at his pocket calendar. "Could we make it early in the morning, say 7 a.m. ?"

"I think that would be fine," said Dr. Sharp. "Go to the information desk in the main lobby, and they'll give you directions to my office."

"Who was that on the phone?" inquired Carol as she came into the Humbleton family room.

"My next quest," said Harry. "I'm going to visit next week with Dr. Charlie Sharp, and talk about control."

"Control is one thing you know a lot about," said Carol. "Harry, I have reservations about this search. I wonder if this is your mid-life crisis starting early. Shouldn't we just let sleeping dogs lie?"

"I don't think I could if I wanted to," said Harry, picking up a medical journal. "I really feel like I have to go forward."

"Well, as I said, you've been in a good mood recently. You don't act like a person in crisis."

"How does a person in crisis look?" asked Harry.

"More frazzled than you are."

Harry picked up his journal, and began to turn pages frantically, shaking the leaves as he went. "Frazzled, who's frazzled?" They both laughed.

The next Thursday, Harry again got up early and drove to Summit General. He got directions to Dr. Sharp's office and took the elevator upstairs. The office window looked out to the East where the morning sun was just driving away the night clouds. Dr. Sharp was tall and angular, his frame fitting his name. He had thick wiry hair, salt and pepper in color. His eyes were dark brown and his nose hawk like. His thin neck protruded from a scrub suit top worn beneath a long white lab coat. His hands were thrust into his pockets. He looked like a senior surgeon.

But his eyes were soft, and his cheeks were rosy, giving him an informal cast that contrasted with his angular chin and neck. Dr. Sharp went right to the agenda of the meeting, almost continuing the telephone conversation.

"Medical training emphasizes the need to control the environment. Surgical training is the most extreme example of this. Certainly it's essential that a surgeon have control of bleeding, and of his wound, and the care related to what he has done. With the same token, any doctor who prescribes a treatment for a patient has to have authority proportionate to the responsibility.

"But the medical profession goes beyond that. Medical students are left brained. So arc the members of the medical school admissions committees, the faculty, and the clinical teachers. This reinforces whatever personality tendencies exist in the entering students and creates a very rigid phalanx of mature professionals."

"That's a pretty strong indictment," said Harry. "I think that what you're calling need to control, I would simply

call the strong personality needed to deal with quick decisions on life and death matters."

"Point conceded. But it goes beyond that. In most areas
of human activity, an excess of a strength becomes a
weakness, a tragic flaw."

He began to pace about the well-appointed office. "Let
me distinguish between leading and dominating. Leaders
see where things need to go. They use persuasive skills to
share that vision with colleagues. In a hierarchical organization, they may even tell subordinates what they want.
But, they'll almost always do better, if they let the subordinates work out exactly how to achieve the goal. They
don't need to tell them how to do it.

"The person intent on dominating, however, has to control the process. He somehow feels it isn't done right if it
doesn't have his stamp every inch of the way. This not
only disparages the intelligence and resourcefulness of
colleagues, it throws a tremendous burden on the shoulders of the one dominating.

"When a person is totally focused on a goal, and insists
on being in charge, that person becomes one sided. And in
time he or she burns out, to use a popular term."

Harry raised his arms and interjected, "Now wait a
minute. I'm not so sure I agree with that. The successful
person has to be focused, and dedicated to goals."

"I'm not suggesting one shouldn't be committed to what
he or she is doing. I'm merely pointing out that for compulsive people like doctors and nurses, it's easy to go over
the line and become a fanatic.

"Furthermore, there's subtle pleasure in learning to
delegate," he went on. "People are complex, diseases are
complex, and healing is complex. Involving more than one

person ensures a higher chance of success. It also makes the process more interesting, and more fun. I'm certain it can actually be done with less total energy expended.

"Whenever you let others tap into their own spirit for solutions to problems, you get more output per unit input. It took me a while to learn that. I was past my residency and a staff surgeon before I saw how much energy I was wasting trying to make people do things my way."

Sharp looked up and pointed toward the wall where a plaque was displayed. It said "More output per input."

"People think that they become more efficient by blanking out other thoughts from their heads as they pursue some target," he said. "To an extent that's true. But intensity can be the father of isolation.

"Unfortunately, even though our profession makes a big fuss over consultations and teamwork, the truth is that we physicians are trained to act and decide independently. We're naive about the meaning of collaboration. We're like a professional baseball team with a collection of superstars, each one thinking he's the best athlete of the century. Many of those teams don't do well, because the big egos and the financial rewards discourage them from sacrifice bunts, or swinging for a hit and run. Collaboration is terribly important, not just because it's necessary for effectiveness, but because it forces balance."

"I'm not sure I follow that," said Harry as he cocked his eyebrow skeptically.

"Let me put it this way. Have you read profiles of doctors, or politicians, or executives, who have achieved some huge goal? When you study them and their methods, what emerges is their ability to focus and concentrate. Life is like one of those guns and butter curves you learned in freshman economics. The more resources you put into guns, the less you have to make butter, and vice versa. The more one puts into a career, the less is available for other activities, such as pleasure, or relationships with others.

"Something always has to give. There's no way to achieve extraordinary success in one area of living, without sacrificing something else. And real living means balancing. Aristotle noted that twenty-four hundred years ago. I think we in medicine, having come to value scientific achievement so much, have created a culture that's out of balance."

"Being a doctor is like walking a tight rope," said Harry. "I understand how we can get so wrapped up in our work that we forget about other things. After all, what we do isn't just important work, it's interesting."

"So are lots of things in life. Part of it is where we place our values. But part of it's merely opening our eyes to see things broadly. And I submit that our medical culture discourages that kind of introspection. That's all."

"Okay, here I agree with you," said Harry. "When we work so hard, we lose time for reflection about the meaning of what we do. Part of my need is to put that into perspective."

Sharp nodded and resumed. "What we do, taking care of sick people, becomes so much a part of our self identity, that we lose perspective. Think of it this way: Suppose you couldn't be a doctor any more. Where would you be? What would be your idea of your worth as a human? Where else would you fit?"

Sharp stopped momentarily, while Harry pondered the question. Then he answered himself. "Only when we can think of ourselves without our medical clothing can we begin to have a framework for viewing things in perspective. Besides, what are we to do if the rewards we thought we had from being a doctor stop? Are we then just an empty instrument bag? That's why doctors are depressed now. Things are changing, and they aren't getting all the rewards from practice they think they should. And so they're glum. I'm saying, look up and look out. Stop trying to control and dominate. It's a formula for frustration and failure."

"You really feel strongly about this, don't you?" said Harry, stopping to let the passion of Dr. Sharp's remarks sink in.

"I sure do. I got these gray hairs doing a lot of reflecting, and I'm convinced these insights are as valuable to our younger colleagues as teaching them new operations."

"You know, you should come to lunch with me and Bill Stokes. He and I have been meeting for years, on the fourth Friday of every month, and we talk about balancing. Bill's really a master balancer. Do you know him?"

"No, though I have read some of his articles. He's an internist, isn't he?"

"Bill's not just an internist. He's a father, a husband, a painter, and he plays baseball in a league for men over fifty-five. He and I occasionally include an outside guest at our lunch meetings. I think he'd be happy to share some of his balancing skills. Sometimes I share my theories on non-control with acquaintances of his. Let me call him, and why don't you plan to have lunch with us two weeks from Friday?"

"Sounds fine to me," said Harry. "I think I've taken enough of your time for now. Let me go home and reflect on some of these thoughts. I wish I had been taking notes. You were dropping the pearls right and left there."

"I don't know how many of them are pearls, and how many are sand particles in the eyes," laughed Dr. Sharp. "Don't get too compulsive. If I can draw you some new ways of seeing things, it's time well spent. I'll see you later."

Harry left Dr. Sharp, and walked out of his office with a spring in his step. Where have these people been he wondered. Why haven't we heard from them louder? Or are they there all the time, and as he says, we need to rub the sand out of our eyes.

Dr. Sharp's voice echoed in his mind: When you let others tap into their own spirit for solutions to problems, you get more output per unit input.

*          *          *          *          *

# Chapter 8.

# *Mastering Balance*

**O**ver the next two weeks, Harry went about the tasks of his practice with a certain optimism he hadn't experienced in months. Many of the frustrating patients didn't seem so frustrating any more. He saw his colleagues in a different light. He read the indignant letters to the editors of the medical journals expressing anger at all the changes in medicine. He saw through the language of the letters into the spirit of the writers. He saw the unreal expectations. And he was saddened.

The day before the scheduled meeting with Drs. Sharp and Stokes, he called Dr. Sharp's office to verify the time and place of the meeting. That morning, he made sure he stayed on schedule in the office.

He didn't know Dr. Stokes personally, and so he asked his associates if anyone knew him. Several said they had been impressed with his commentaries in the medical society magazine. A couple had been on panels with him for the state Society of Internal Medicine. All portrayed him as a cerebral, but highly practical, physician.

When the three doctors assembled for their meeting at a small Mexican restaurant in the central part of the city, Harry immediately relaxed with Dr. Stokes' manner. Stokes' bio in the medical society roster listed his age at fifty-seven, but he looked closer to forty-five. He had brown hair with gray temples, and brown eyebrows, below which gazed the most penetrating blue eyes Harry had ever encountered. They seemed to fix on whoever was speaking, like a camera lens, or a video camera, seeing and recording everything in view.

Stokes greeted Harry. "Glad to have you with us. Charlie occasionally brings other 'insight seekers' to these lunches. We're all the richer for what we learn from one another."

Sharp briefed Stokes on how Harry came to him, and Stokes chuckled in that same knowing way as Leslie Ladd and Len Spector. Harry suspected all were protégés of Sanford Hayworth.

After they ordered, Stokes began. "Usually we talk about some contemporary issue. Medical is okay, but not clinical. Those are the ground rules. Today, since we have you with us, we'll put aside the usual format. Let's talk in more general terms."

"Dr. Sharp portrayed you as the master balancer." said Harry. "He claimed you have a formula for managing time that lets you achieve a lot but also keep a perspective on living as a citizen and a human."

Stokes appeared to wince, and shrugged his shoulders apologetically. "I'm flattered. I'm not anything that special. I'm just lucky to have a good wife, and a religion that has given me a philosophy on caring for self and the world.

"When I got into medicine, and saw how demanding clinical practice was going to be, I had a little mini-crisis of the soul. I had invested years in school and residency. I was married and had a new baby. I wasn't sure how to live up to all my responsibilities.

"Something had to suffer. Patients always got first claim on my time. My wife started to resent that. I was angry. I wanted to see my children grow up. I also enjoyed sports.

I really believe in that old Roman adage, 'mens sana in corpore sano'"

"I remember that from high school Latin," responded Harry. "A sound mind in a sound body."

"You know it," said Stokes. "Nothing new there. Articulated two thousand years ago in Italy. Really known by all cultures if you study it."

Harry noted Stokes spoke in short declarative sentences. It was as though he wanted to keep each thought distinct to make an impact on the listener.

Stokes picked up a spoon, and held it by the bowl, as though the handle was a pointer. "Balance comes from realism. Realism comes from self-awareness. Self-awareness comes from self-care. Self-care starts with self-assessment.

"We may be dealing with patients, our families, or our inner selves. We have to seek realistic objectives. We have to know the end point of what we are doing, and what outcomes we can expect. We can't do that intelligently unless we start by understanding ourselves.

"I'm a real believer in introspection. I preach it to other MD's, because, for a group as collectively bright as physicians are, we're clueless about the meaning of what we do. Collaboration with others is the way to keep life in balance. Do you remember 'Samuel Shem'?"

"Sure," said Harry. 'The House of God'; an irreverent review of life as a young physician in training."

"That's the one," said Stokes. "He made the point that medicine is part of life, not vice versa. We sometimes get so caught up in what we do as doctors that we forget that."

Stokes had the floor, and for all his directness, Harry could see he was getting into high gear, and loved the histrionics of performing, even to an audience of two. "My avowed goal is to live and preach balance. That's why I play baseball. I know it's frivolous for a bunch of middle aged arthritics to get out there and act like kids. But it not only gives us exercise and keeps us young, it keeps us doing inconsequential things. And that's important. We doctors take living pretty seriously. We see so much sickness, we can come to see existence as heavier than the Creator intended it to be."

"I do understand that," interjected Harry. "I used to take golf lessons from an old pro who taught a lot of doctors and lawyers. He said that he thought the reason so many doctors play golf is that it requires them to think about something different for several hours."

Stokes chimed in, putting down the teaspoon he had been waving. "I think it's more than that. Use golf as the illustration instead of baseball. This doesn't relate only to doctors. It applies to anyone who has responsibilities, and has to concentrate and focus in his or her everyday work. I think it's precisely being preoccupied with trivial things like where the ball is going that's the benefit. I know there are many things that attract people to golf; walking, being outdoors, being with friends, the wager. But mostly, it's concentrating on things that really don't matter much. No one's life depends on whether the ball is hit straight. No one's survival depends on whether the hole is uphill, or whether the wind is blowing toward or away from the flight of the ball."

He picked up the spoon again, and balanced the handle on his extended index finger. He gestured toward the wavering utensil. "There's even more than that to this idea of balance. It relates to being a part of, rather than resisting, change. Look at this spoon perched on my finger."

He moved the spoon slightly, and it toppled off. He picked it up, and placed it over two fingers. He moved it again, but the spoon remained stationary. "I know I have many sources of support; my wife, my children, my church, my profession, my friends. Because I have such a wide range of support, I don't have to fear change. I can step out to meet it. That makes me more effective professionally. Just like the spoon can better resist being knocked off when it has two supports instead of one."

"That's a different point of view for a doctor," said Harry. "Most of us tend to hate change exactly because it's unpredictable. We like to be in charge and immutable."

"Well, it shouldn't be that way," said Dr. Stokes, taking a big bite out of a rolled tortilla. "Let's finish our lunch and pay the bill. I have to get back to the office, and I suspect, so do both of you."

Harry looked at his watch. An hour and a half had elapsed, and he hadn't been aware of it. He had been so engrossed in Stokes' ideas, he had nearly forgotten to eat his own lunch. He quickly finished his portion, and they walked out of the restaurant.

"Well, I hope these ideas help you," said Bill Stokes. "I don't want to leave you thinking I'm blasé about responsibility. In fact, I think having balance has helped me to be a more caring physician."

"I won't dispute that," said Harry.

Charlie Sharp spoke up at that point. "I told you he'd give you valuable insights, Harry. We're going to call you the sage of the spoon, Bill."

Dr. Sharp returned to the table to leave a tip, and Stokes looked at Harry. "There's another person you should talk to on caring and how it relates to making medicine part of life rather than making life subservient to practicing medicine. Do you know Don Walters?"

"Of course," said Harry. "He's on the staff at Memorial with me. A fine neurologist. Has lots of patients with multiple sclerosis. I don't know how he keeps his cheerful side, given how sick his patients are."

"That's exactly why I think you'd benefit from talking with him," said Dr. Stokes. "He knows more than anyone I know about the importance of caring. Give him a call when you have the time."

"Thanks, I will," said Harry, and they shook hands.

That night as he was falling asleep, he kept repeating to himself. Balance comes from realism. Realism comes from self- awareness. Self-awareness comes from self-care. Self-care starts with self-assessment. Balance is easier with a broad base of support.

*        *        *        *        *

# Chapter 9.

# *Caring about Care*

**H**arry dreamed about the string that night. He tried to stiffen the string with glue. But then the string stuck to the tabletop, and still buckled. He lubricated the surface with silicone spray, but that didn't work either. The string slithered and looped more than ever. Hayworth held out his hand, and kept repeating, "Come to this end and pull, Harry." But Harry couldn't move. He felt like he was constrained by a rope made of the very string he was trying to push.

The next day he saw Don Walters at Memorial Hospital. Walters was youthful looking, though in his mid-fifties. He was stocky in build, with no neck, and a jolly chin that sat right on his collar. He walked jauntily and affected plaid sport coats. Sometimes he wore a bow tie. His colleagues considered him a bit of a character. Harry cornered him in the coffee lounge. "I had lunch yesterday with Bill Stokes. We talked about balance. He did the spoon trick. Suggested I ask you about your formula for caring.

"I must admit, Don, I've often wondered what's the secret? How do you manage to remain so upbeat? I've seen you a hundred times, talking to families of patients with terminal wasting diseases, and you always seem to be able to mount a positive outlook. What are you on?"

"Nothing chemical," replied Walters. "That's a complicated question. I don't think I can give you a short answer. If you've had an encounter with Bill Stokes, I need to go into a little depth. I'm not as quick with examples and illustrations as he is. If I have a secret it's more my reaction to my childhood than any formal system. Come on down to the EEG lab after I read this morning's tracings, and I'd be happy to talk with you."

"Sounds fair," said Harry. "I have three patients to see. How long will it take you to finish in the lab?"

"Probably an hour."

"Good, I'll see you at the EEG lab in an hour," said Harry, and he turned to head for the elevator.

He went to radiology, checked his patients' x-rays, and walked upstairs to make rounds. His mind was as much on Don Walters, as on his patients. But he found himself being optimistic, even jocular, with them. Maybe Walters was exerting some subtle influence by remote control.

An hour later, he went to the basement of the hospital, where the neuro-diagnostic laboratory was situated. There, in the windowless room, amidst pages of incomprehensible squiggles, he found Don Walters busily flipping through sheets of paper.

"Glad to take a break," said Walters. "Let me finish this dictation. It's the last report. Then I can take some time with you."

With that he picked up his recording microphone and began to drone with the scientific detachment of the experienced neurologist. When he had finished, he took out a plate of pastries and poured a cup of coffee for both of them. Then he began.

"I guess Mother Nature just gave me the right balance of hormones," he said, bisecting a blueberry muffin with a stainless steel table knife. "I know what you're wondering, how can I stand day after day to be in a field where most of the patients have inexorable lethal diseases? Probably my attitude comes from when I was growing up."

Walters halved another muffin, and offered a portion to Harry. Harry raised his palm to decline and said, "Thanks, coffee's enough for me right now."

Walters went on. "My older brother had muscular dystrophy, and I watched him waste away. Mom and Dad were so good about taking care of him that it seemed natural for me and my younger sister to help in his care.

"In addition, sometimes, when I was alone, in the quiet of the night, I'd become introspective. Why did my brother get sick, but my sister and I didn't? It wasn't his fault. It wasn't anything she or I had done. It was just one of those imponderables. I either had to become a fatalist, or seek some meaning in suffering."

"As time went on, I thought it might be a good idea to become a doctor. When I graduated, going into neurology just kind of followed. I never even gave it a thought. By then my brother had died, but my mother and father were still alive, and I very much respected how they had taken care of him. And my dad, who was about as gruff and matter of fact as they make 'em, was always there for my brother. Both my parents seemed to know that life has positives and negatives, and that our role as humans is to make things better for those with whom we come in contact. And if we can have some fun, or make enough money to be comfortable, that's a bonus. But it's that caring for the other person that makes the difference.

Harry had a mental flashback to Mel Filipone the barber.

"Now, don't over-read what I say," went on Dr. Walters. "I'm no saint. I'll confess, sometimes caring for a person with a fatal illness really becomes too much to handle.

"For some reason, I've seen a lot of doctors as patients over the years. Some with strokes, some with MS and a couple with Lou Gehrig's disease. You know what a sick doctor appreciates more than anything else? A colleague that cares about him or her. That's much more important than technical knowledge."

"You must have developed some way of saying farewell to patients," said Harry. "What's your philosophy there?"

Walters put his thumb to his chin pensively. "I don't have any strict approach," he said. "I do have a conviction that we doctors need to learn how to say good-bye to our patients.

"In medical school we're taught to interview patients, how to get their past histories and develop rapport with them. In time, we get good at it and can do it pretty fast.

"But, we don't have classes in how to say good-bye to dying patients. None of us likes it. Some of us never learn to do it, and we either go into some specialty where we don't have to deal with the dying, or we avoid it. Then we really do a disservice to our patients."

Walters slowed down, and looked directly into Harry's face. "I knew someplace along the way that I was good at saying good-bye. It wasn't that it didn't hurt me as much as the next person. It was just that from my experience with my brother, I had learned to face into a person's suffering. I know this sounds heavy, and I try not to dwell on it. But this is my operating philosophy," he said, shrugging his shoulders.

"Another point, that I read somewhere," he continued, "is that we caregivers have to speak out about suffering, for our own humanity. Otherwise we bottle it up, and it eats us.

Harry felt compelled to make a joke. "You don't pop Prozac every day?"

Don Walters laughed. "No, but some of us probably should. As I said a minute ago, I think Nature gave me a good supply of endorphins, or some hormone that sustains me. Maybe it's simply optimism. Do you know Mike Curran?"

"Somewhat," said Harry. "He's a new neurologist on the staff, isn't he?"

"Right. He got angry at me one day last month. He was annoyed that I keep an upbeat attitude with all the calamities in the world. He was frustrated and said 'Walters, I know why you're so damned optimistic. It's because you went to college in the Eisenhower era. You're a product of the 50's.' I don't know if Eisenhower, or the 50's have anything to do with it, but I've always been lucky enough to see the part of the glass that's full.

"The neurological patients with their muscle wasting, and their spasticity, are vulnerable humans. And I care about them. It's no more complex than that. I wish I could explain my thinking more, but I really can't."

Harry was moved by Walters' simplicity and lack of self-consciousness. Harry was silent for a moment, and then said, "I think I understand you. For some of us, being able to see the optimistic side is as much a gift as a musical car, or athletic coordination. Often, the gifted athlete can't explain how he does what he does. His sense of balance just tells him where the parts of his body need to be."

"Yes, but some athletes can coach and teach others. That's a gift, too. They don't just feel, they understand."

"That's what I mean," said Harry. "Can you explain what makes you able to stay caring and optimistic?"

Walters paused, and the smile left his face. Uncharacteristically, he became silent. "It's just a matter of concern," he finally explained. "Look, it's pretty easy to be concerned about one's brother, like I was when I was a child. It's a matter of seeing other people who aren't your friends or relatives as having the same feelings and aspirations you do. It's a matter of identifying, I guess."

"Don't you become morose, then, if you think, 'This could happen to me'?"

"Not really," replied Don Walters. "I don't understand why there's suffering and pain in the world. They're mysteries. I know there's some directing force that allows good and bad to happen. Call it God, call it whatever you want. It exists as surely as the sun and the moon. I didn't make the world, but my task is to improve it. Maybe only a tiny bit. Maybe only temporarily. Maybe it'll be futile. But that's my philosophy, and it makes it easier to deal with sick people."

Harry thanked Don Walters. "Don, I'm impressed. I wish more of us could understand our roles the way you expressed it. I don't mean just doctors and nurses. Wouldn't it be great if families of patients could have that benefit? Have you ever thought of working these ideas into a speech, or writing an article?"

"Yes, from time to time I have," replied Walters. "The trouble is these thoughts are private. I can say them comfortably to someone I know like you. I don't know if I'm up to being an evangelist."

"Think about it," said Harry, and he left the lab.

That afternoon Harry decided to call Sanford Hayworth, his mentor. As he mentally composed what he would say, he thought back to Don Walters' message. We need to learn to say both hello and good-bye to those we care for.

        \*        \*        \*        \*

# Chapter 10.

# *Going Beyond Training*

**H**arry could feel spring in the air as he returned to his office from Memorial Hospital. There were new leaves on the trees, not lush enough to make the branches wave, but green enough to replace the gray branches of winter. Outside his office building iris and tulips were sprouting from the chilly soil. Harry felt rejuvenated.

That afternoon, after he had finished seeing his patients, Harry phoned Sanford Hayworth.

"It's about time for me to check in with a progress report," he began. "I've been all over the county. I feel like a newspaper reporter gathering background for a story."

"In a sense, that's right," said the voice at the other end of the receiver. "You're learning how your own autobiography might go. It may never be put down in actual words, but I'm sure your internal dialogue could be put into book form."

"I've visited a listening dermatologist, a pathologist who hates to be perfect, an anti-control surgeon, an internist preoccupied with balance, and an optimistic neurologist. Now that's a menagerie if there ever was one."

Hayworth then quizzed him. "Have you learned from them?"

"Definitely. Each of them had some particular insight, some particular trait he or she uses as a guidepost."

"Good, that's what I hoped you'd say. Well, what do you want to do next?"

"Is there more?" asked Harry.

"Oh, yes," replied the older man. "Actually, we can learn from almost everyone we meet. You've seen people that I knew would be sources of inspiration."

He laughed. "I have more. Does the name Andrew Runyon mean anything to you?"

"Of course," said Harry. "Professor of Medicine at University Medical Center. The first African American graduate of the combined M. D.-Ph. D. program at the University. Former Dean at Cal, the force behind that experimental curriculum they're using."

"A visionary," agreed Hayworth. "We began to correspond on some of these human issues several years ago when we happened to sit next to each other at a banquet for the American College.

"Even though he earned his academic stripes with brilliant research on arteriosclerosis, he got interested in prevention of diseases, and then in getting doctors to balance technology with human understanding.

"If I had to characterize Andrew Runyon, I'd call him one of the most creative people ever to earn an M. D. Go talk with him, and I think he'll add to your experience."

"That may take a while," said Harry. "University Medical Center is two hundred miles away. I'd have to take a whole day off. Do you think it would really benefit me that much?"

"Absolutely. We're all products of medical education. The conforming period, the training, these shaped our views and taught us to put our profession first. Andrew Runyon has grown beyond that. His writings indicate it. In addition to being a persuasive speaker, he has an engaging personality."

Harry knew he'd best concede. "Okay. You've given me a lot of help so far. I guess I can stay with it through Dr. Runyon."

And so, he called Andrew Runyon's office at University Medical Center and requested an appointment with the illustrious professor. It was three weeks before Runyon could get the time free, which was good, because it permitted Harry to arrange time away from the office and get coverage while he would be gone.

Carol was perplexed by this pilgrimage, but she saw Harry changing, and she liked the changes, and so she urged him to go.

It took Harry a full half-day to reach University Medical Center. The trees along the interstate were green, and spring grass speckled the fields of the farms and orchards. It was a delightful drive, marred only by having to spend the last hour snaking bumper to bumper through the innards of the metropolis where the medical Mecca was located.

The University Medical Center was beautiful. Red brick with an old fashioned eastern appearance, it had an avant garde cantilevered construction, clearly a blend of tradition and innovation. Dr. Runyon's office was in the outpatient wing, which was only three stories high and more humble looking. It had obviously had been the first building on the medical campus.

Runyon's office was spacious, reflecting his senior status, and the age of the building. It had two floor length windows that looked out on a sloping terrace toward an ultra-modern laboratory complex. The furniture was a blend of wood and steel, with bound journals and textbooks everywhere. A Pentium equipped Compaq computer with speakers, CD-ROM attachment, and a laser printer signified this was not the lair of some old fogy professor, but an active academic.

Dr. Runyon fit with his office. He was in person also a blend of the traditional and the innovative. He had steel wool gray hair trimmed short, and wore a conservative, button-down shirt. However, he sported a wild tie and he spoke like someone who was thirty, rather than sixty.

"Glad to see you," Runyon said, greeting Harry. "I got a call about you. Your friend, Sanford really respects you. Say hello for me when you get back home."

Harry opened the conversation. "I've been on a pilgrimage the past few months. I was burning out on the practice of medicine. I knew Dr. Hayworth and his reputation in our area as an advisor. I asked him for suggestions on how to rekindle that spirit. You're among the various people he suggested I consult. I understand your work here at University Medical Center has helped practitioners as well as trainees see where the profession fits in their lives."

"I'm flattered," returned Runyon. "Yes, I'm proud not only of what we're doing for medical students and house officers, but what we're doing for our alumni, and for that matter, practicing physicians all over the state, regardless of where they trained."

He swung back in his desk chair. "There are major changes under way in medical education. We have a rich legacy from the scientist-clinicians of the early part of this century, but we've gone so far toward science, we sometimes forget medicine involves applying science to sick people.

"Applicants to medical school tend to be cerebral. They're usually idealistic youngsters who excel at science and see medicine as an uplifting way to use science for the benefit of people. That's a noble idea, and we can't afford to dilute or squelch it."

The afternoon sun beamed in on Runyon's desk. Harry saw fluttering shadows from an oak tree outside the window. A noble tree, and a noble idea. Runyon continued. "On the other hand, the primary goal of universities is the advancement of knowledge, not taking care of the sick. Faculty members have tended to emphasize science and disease so much that the human elements have been submerged.

"Ever since the nineteen-fifties, when the federal government chose to support medical schools by funding research, the pendulum has swung way toward science and the study of diseases.

"Education can give skills, but it can't guarantee a compassionate outlook. We've produced a goodly number of highly skilled medical technicians. Most practicing physicians sense this along the way, and unlearn the rigid scientific scrutiny they received in medical school."

Through the other long window, Harry could see the blue green of a spruce tree. He thought to himself what a choice spot for reflection Andrew Runyon enjoyed. "Besides the preoccupation with science and data, medical training is depersonalizing. There's a lot of hazing involved. 'If you want to be a doctor, you have to be tough, like me' goes the philosophy."

"Tell me about it," said Harry. "

"Yes, unfortunately, most of us had similar experiences during training. That's what I mean. Someplace along the way, with the hassling and the demeaning, those idealistic young scientists metamorphose into cynics.

"Fortunately, most mature physicians come to see this, and grow beyond it. But some don't and remain defensive all their careers. They're embarrassed if they aren't perfect, and they become arrogant. That's the public stereotype of physicians today: arrogant. It leads to the idea that we alone know what is best for people. We're seeing the down side of that. Its best form is paternalism, but its dark side is arrogance."

"What's the remedy?" asked Harry.

"First is understanding," said Runyon. "No one consciously wants to be arrogant. It's a big step forward just to see how the perfectionism of medical training makes it difficult to acknowledge mistakes. The culture teaches by fear, and arrogance is a defense against that fear.

"In addition, the insightful and effective physician knows how to listen. The person trying to be perfect tends to be insecure and self-centered. That person isn't a good listener. That's why many MD's aren't good listeners. It's not just because they're in a hurry."

Harry looked at Runyon, and again glanced out at the oak and spruce outside the window. Both examples of organisms steadfast but adaptable, he thought.

Runyon said proudly, "This is one of the real advances in our curriculum here at University Medical Center. We're teaching our medical students to listen, to see the patients in their own environment. A by-product of this is that the student physicians learn to use their own feelings as diagnostic tools. Many mature practicing physicians have unconsciously learned to do this."

"Yes, I know what you mean by that," said Harry nodding his head in agreement. "When I have a depressed patient, I tend to feel either anxious or depressed myself.

When I get an uneasy feeling, I know either the patient isn't telling me the whole story, or is manipulating me in some way. Being aware of this has made me a better history taker, and a better physician."

"Then you already know what I mean. That's what I'm talking about when I say a person has to grow beyond being a body technician to become a physician. For professors like me, the trick is to be human enough to be good role models.

"Many professors think if they have encyclopedic knowledge, and are up on the latest literature, they can bamboozle medical students and interns. It just doesn't work that way. Medical students are bright. They can tell a fraud. They need role models who are human.

"That's another thing we're excited about here at University Medical Center," commented Runyon. "Educating physicians in the humanities. You know a steady diet of science may lead to brilliant understanding of diseases, but it isn't the way to be a good physician. We require courses in literature and history during the premedical years, plus have medical humanities during the four years of medical school.

Harry leaned backward in his chair. "That's all fine," he said, "but my experience suggests you can talk about humanism, and educate in the humanities as long as you want, but that doesn't guarantee humanistic behavior."

"Point accepted," said Runyon. "That's why we work to hire a faculty that's insightful. And let me tell you, given the competing requirements to teach cell biology, and immunology, that's a tall order.

"I can see you're already a true physician. You wouldn't even be here if you were content as a body technician. That's another frustrating thing. The people who need to broaden their outlook the most are the most difficult to reach."

"That's not confined to medical education, Dr. Runyon," said Harry. "It's the reverse of preaching to the choir."

"I'm afraid so."

The shadows were getting longer. The breeze had subsided, and the oak leaves were still. The room was momentarily still. "I've enjoyed discussing these things with you," commented Runyon. "You're already insightful. You wouldn't like to leave your practice and come join our faculty, would you?"

"Thanks for the compliment," said Harry. "If I could get an office this peaceful and comfortable, I might consider it. I think my destiny is to be a practitioner more than a teacher or investigator. But it's helpful to think about how medical training influences our medical culture, and how sometimes we have to unlearn what we've been taught."

"It won't stop," said Runyon. "That's the nature of it. We learn, and then we learn more deeply. Sometimes that means unlearning, and sometimes it just means peeling the onion another layer. It depends on how you want to see it."

Harry looked up at a clock on Runyon's bookshelf. He had to leave if he hoped to get back home that night. Runyon asked, "Do you know Nancy Rudolph? She lives in your city."

"By name," said Harry. "She teaches nursing classes at our hospital. Very dynamic lady, I'm told. The word is she's revamping nursing education."

"Correct," said Runyon. "You might give her a call when you get home. She spent some time with me helping design our curriculum. Since she lives near you, I think she'd be willing to give you still different insights.

"But my thoughts for you are, revel in being human and work on sensitizing yourself to feelings as a diagnostic tool. Then you'll continue to be a credit to us at University."

Runyon escorted Harry to the elevator. "Give my best to Sandy the sage back there, and call me if I can help you in any other ways." He turned back toward his office, his stethoscope jingling in his pocket as he walked.

What a role model for the medical students, thought Harry to himself. On the drive home that evening, he kept repeating what he learned from Andrew Runyon: Unlearn what was depersonalizing; revel in being human; use your feelings as a diagnostic tool. Grow beyond being a technician to become a healer.

\*       \*       \*       \*       \*

# Chapter 11.

# Confessions of a Redhead

**H**arry was very busy with his practice the next week. But he didn't feel busy. He went through his hospital rounds with recovered energy. His patients seemed more interesting than ever. He wasn't sure if he was just hitting a wave of challenging cases, or whether he was seeing the same patients in a different way. Whatever it was, he was enjoying his practice more.

He called Sanford Hayworth to brief him on the visit to Dr. Runyon. "And he wanted me to be sure to say hello to you on his behalf."

"Runyon's a good man." said Hayworth. "Wish we had more academicians like him. We'd have broader and better practitioners."

"Have you heard of Nancy Rudolph?"

"Yes," said the older man. "Did Runyon tell you about her? I heard she helped him design some of his curriculum."

"He said she's doing some remarkable things in teaching nurses new ways to think, and that I could learn from her."

"Why don't we both visit her?" replied the senior physician. "I only know of her work in a general way, and I'd like to learn too."

"I'll look her up and ask if she'll share some of her ideas with both of us," volunteered Harry.

Hayworth chuckled. "This is good. You're getting to see diverse viewpoints. I'd like to think these people are representative, and not totally eclectic. I think they're role models for us, regardless of our work, and I do think we all need to mentor one another."

As soon as Harry hung up the telephone, he looked up the number of Northside Memorial Health Center, where Nancy Rudolph was Vice President of Nursing Services. He dialed her office, and was put through to her secretary.

"Ms. Rudolph loves to talk about the work she's doing," said the secretary. "She's an evangelist. She's busy, and so she may not be able to give a lot of time. You know nurses have been coming from all over the country to pick her brain. She says she wishes she had a twin sister. Let me ask her to call you, because she likes to make her own appointments for informal visits like this."

That evening, Harry got a call from Nancy Rudolph. He could hear her enthusiasm through the phone wires.

He opened the conversation. "Dr. Andrew Runyon at the University Center said you're reworking nursing philosophy, and that you might share some of your ideas.

"Sharing ideas with M.D.'s is always fun for me," said Nancy Rudolph. "It's often a challenge. When do you want to meet?"

Harry looked at his calendar, and gave her some dates. They picked the following Friday, and decided to meet at her office at 4 p.m. "You won't mind if I bring a friend along, I hope. His name is Sanford Hayworth. He's been interested in better ways of taking care of people and communication between nurses and doctors." Harry didn't know the latter for certain, but he figured Hayworth could qualify for that description. It might make Nancy Rudolph interested in them.

"Oh, yes, I know of some of his projects. I've seen them profiled in the Sunday paper. I'd love to talk with him," said Nancy Rudolph.

I guess Sanford Hayworth didn't need me to boost his stock with her, thought Harry, chagrined at his ingratiating impulse.

The following Friday, the two doctors went to Nancy Rudolph's office at Northside. They exchanged handshakes, and sat down. She was tall, thin, and had a shock of auburn hair flecked with gray, that looked too variegate to be dyed. Her name fit her hair. Her cheeks and arms were freckled. Her eyes were green. She wore a green suit and blouse that complemented her skin coloring perfectly. She radiated cool energy.

A striking figure, thought Harry as he looked at her. Her eyes caught his, and he felt embarrassed for staring. She smiled and Harry thought she sensed his look, but appreciated it as a compliment.

"Glad you both could come," began Nancy. "What can I do for you?"

"Well, we were told you've been teaching your nurses different ways of seeing their patients," Harry responded. "We're trying to develop a system to see our patients differently too, and we're interested in your philosophy and what you have accomplished. We're a couple of superannuated students." He pointed toward his senior associate in the opposite chair as he tried vainly to make a joke.

"We're all students in one way or another," said Nancy Rudolph directly. "I enjoy telling people about my experiences here. When I took over as Director of Nursing at Northside, the thing that struck me the most was how these bright women, both young and old, had been taught in nursing school to be reactive. They seemed to have had the initiative squeezed from them. They had been forced to conform so much that the best ones were leaving direct patient care to do specialized tasks. I saw I had to reverse that trend because our patients nowadays are sicker than ever. A lot of senior citizens live in the neighborhood near Northside."

She gestured as she spoke. Long slender fingers extended dramatically, though her tone was conversational and matter of fact. "I saw myself dealing with intelligent people, mostly women, but a number of men as well, whose culture demanded they react to doctors' orders. Some of these nurses probably are smarter than the doctors, but they kept deferring to the doctors. I decided that inhibits their being the most effective advocates for their patients. I was going to change that, or at least go down swinging if I couldn't change the system.

"Fortunately, Dr. Cecil Hardenback was Chief of Staff when I came on board, and he was broad minded enough to support me. But there were a lot of doctors who were such control freaks they felt threatened by the idea that nurses might actually make suggestions to them, or even worse, tell them what needed to be done for their patients.

She sighed and then frowned. "At the beginning, some of them tried to get me fired by going to the Senior Administrator. Some doctors even used their friendships with members of the Board of Trustees to skewer me. But it didn't work. My husband's Chief of Ob-Gyn at the Clavenger Clinic, in Brook Grove, and too many of the members of the Board knew both of us for their negative lobbying to work."

"Don't tell me Ted Householder is your husband," interjected Sanford Hayworth. "I had him as an intern twenty-five years ago. I knew he was engaged to a nurse. I knew he went into Obstetrics. I never connected you with him. I guess the city's getting so big, and the connections so distant, we don't know about one another's personal lives like we used to."

"Well, I'm the one. We're very connected. Many people don't know we're married because I use my maiden name for my own profession. Besides, I was out of nursing for quite a while when our children were growing up. Now, though, they're independent, and so I'm back at it. Nursing is still my fifth love, after Ted and our three daughters.

"Watching my daughters grow up and go to college was part of what motivated me to teach nursing. It was also one of the main reasons I thought nurses could become more assertive. The young women nowadays are getting first rate educations. Many are going to medical school. There are men becoming nurses. Gender distinctions shouldn't mean that much. It was this kind of thinking that challenged me to remold the Nursing Service here at Northside.

"And fortunately, with Dr. Hardenback's and the Board's support, I was able to hang in there. Plus, I'll have to say that many of those flinty staff MD's who were initially defensive are now my greatest testimonials. Believe it or not, even doctors can change. And when they change, their personalities are usually strong enough that they make good allies."

"So what's the formula?" asked Harry.

"I think it's based on twin virtues," replied Nancy Rudolph. "Accountability and trust. We're committed to letting the people closest to the patient make as many of the decisions as possible. We expect the nurses to back up one another, likewise the physical therapists, respiratory therapists, medical technologists, pharmacists, and everyone else. We include the hospital engineers in our meetings, also the billing clerks, and the people who clean the rooms. When representatives are elected from some constituency in the hospital, we expect them to be accountable. They're responsible to get input from their area and speak up.

"The flip side of that is trust. If someone represents a group in a particular project or task force, everyone has to trust that person will really represent their viewpoint."

Harry and Sanford Hayworth nodded understandingly. Nancy Rudolph paused and pushed a gold bracelet back over her wrist.

"When our people deal with the doctors, they can be quite assertive, because they know their stuff. If a nurse calls the doctor at ten P.M. because a patient is short of breath, the doctor knows that the respiratory therapist has also evaluated that patient, and the doctor is going to get ideas on the cause of the shortness of breath, and likely suggestions on what might help solve the problem.

"The nurses know the latest clinical data on their patients, and with on-line information, they can update the doctors quickly. The doctors respect the staff, and the staff respects one another. Everyone's accountable, and trusted.

"It sounds idealistic, but it works. We have very high scores on our patient satisfaction surveys, and our outcomes are as good as the best."

"At Community we've been trying to focus on our patients that way, too," said Hayworth. "You know the clichés about patient focused care. It's been tough, because the organization has been run from the top down, and we've only had partial success in breaking down employees' fear.

"Accountability and trust," he mused. "I hadn't quite framed it that way in my own thinking, but I understand it and I like it. Simple and straightforward."

I've been writing about this notion," said Nancy Rudolph, "and I might even put together a book some day."

"You could call it 'The One Minute Nurse,'" said Harry.

"I'd probably entitle it 'Confessions of a Redhead,'" laughed Nancy. "I hope I've given you gentlemen some ideas to take home with you. If you don't mind, I'm planning to meet Ted for a bike ride. As these spring days get longer, I get more energy."

"Some atavistic response from your Norse gene pool," suggested Hayworth with a smile.

"I haven't analyzed it that much. I just know it's good for a middle-aged lady to be with her man whenever she can. Best of luck to you both." She stood up, shook hands with them, and accompanied them to the parking lot at Northside.

"What a woman," exclaimed Harry as he and his companion walked to their cars.

"Ted Householder was a good natured medical student, well suited for obstetrics. He must have his hands full managing a relationship with that lady," mused Hayworth.

"Shc's vivacious, even passionate," Harry commented as he unlocked the door of his car.

Hayworth looked pensively at Harry, and tapped his ignition key against his index finger. He spoke deliberately. "I have one more person I'd like you to meet."

"I hope he's not in another state. I did benefit from visiting Andrew Runyon up at the university, but I'm not that much of a traveler. I'd like to think in a city as large as ours, we have a complement of original thinkers."

"We do. I'd like to suggest you talk with a woman on the Community Clinic Board with me. She's a retired lawyer who acts as a patient advocate. Her name is Irene Capek."

"A patient advocate. That would round things out, wouldn't it?" said Harry. "You're acquainted with some interesting people. I'll admit I haven't gone wrong yet."

"My office can give you her number," said Sanford Hayworth as he opened the door of his car.

See you later," said Harry as he pulled out of the parking lot. As he headed home, he began to think more about Nancy Rudolph's philosophy: the twin virtues, trust and accountability.

*     *     *     *     *

# Chapter 12.

# The Effective Patient

**H**arry relaxed that weekend. He was off call, and didn't have to go to the hospital, which gave him a chance to visit the farmers' market with Carol and Katie. The warming air of early spring lay over the city, and it seemed all the citizens had adopted the same lazy pace as Harry. He was surprised at how many neighbors he saw buying fruits and vegetables. Strawberries were the delicacy of the day, and Carol made short cake for dessert that night.

On Sunday, the three of them went on a picnic in the hills above the city. They wandered amidst groves of trees, and Katie collected pine cones. Harry lay in bed that evening and wondered how he could create more weekends like this one.

Monday morning he made a telephone call to Irene Capek. A cultured, modulated voice came on the line. "This is Irene," she said, "How may I help you?"

Harry introduced himself as an acquaintance of Sanford Hayworth, and indicated his interest in learning about her work as a patient advocate. The cultured voice became enthusiastic. "By all means, Dr. Humbleton. I would be delighted to meet with you. Sanford Hayworth has been a valuable resource for our group, and occasionally asks me to describe to others how we function. He's rather like the pied piper, you know. One can hardly resist listening to his music. But he benefits people, rather than kidnapping them."

"He certainly has influenced a number of people," Harry returned, as he thumbed the pages of his pocket calendar. "I'm open tomorrow morning. Would it be convenient if I came to your office around ten?" he asked.

"Tomorrow morning at ten would be just fine, Dr. Humbleton. Our name is Help in Healing, and our office is located at 4086 Navajo Road. It's Suite 102. I'll see you then."

Harry hurried to see his hospitalized patients the next morning, so that he could make some extra time for the meeting. He arrived breathless just before ten and looked around for Help in Healing. He found a small sign on an inconspicuous door in the inner courtyard of the office building. He entered a reception area that contained two chairs. Copies of Modern Maturity and The Smithsonian were on a coffee table. A desk was in one corner, and a door led to an inner office. Harry had barely stepped into the suite, when Irene Capek appeared from inside.

Harry thought her to be about sixty-five. Her hair was white with blonde streaks. Her skin was pale, her eyes dark above high cheekbones, her lips thin. She was thick wasted, but trim, and wore a maroon dress. Her jewelry consisted of small gold earrings, a thin gold necklace, and a gold wedding band. She emanated graciousness.

"How do you do, Dr. Humbleton," she began. "I hope you like our office. It's not large, but is very functional.

"Looks fine to me," said Harry politely. "Thanks very much for agreeing to talk with me. Dr. Hayworth has been sending me all over town to meet people who have learned to take what he calls, time out for healing. He uses the expression to mean we all need to stop and take stock of what we're about. I'm assuming you're acquainted with it."

"I've heard him use the term many times. When a doctor or nurse says it, there's a double meaning. But those of us who are not licensed healers often have to engage in the same self-appraisal. Many of our clients here are parents, children, and spouses of people with severe chronic diseases. Sometimes the illnesses ravage the caregivers more than the victims." She paused as she saw Harry nod assent.

"Did Sanford explain my background, and how I got into this?" she asked.

"Not really."

"I escaped from Czechoslovakia as a teen-ager, and managed to get to the United States. I met my husband in college. He went into business, and I went to law school. We married as soon as I graduated, and had a baby right away. So I stayed home, and never practiced. He was involved in international finance, and we traveled to Europe a lot. We had a wonderful life, and were proud of our son. In time, I began to practice family law part time. In that field, an attorney is in many ways a social worker. I helped clients manage their lives, as much as I was their advocate. I came to see how important stable relationships are for families to succeed.

"Our son developed leukemia when he was twenty-five. It was terrible, with bleeding, infections, side effects of chemotherapy, and all that. He died about a year later, not of his disease, but from liver failure brought on by the medicines. We were quite devastated, and for a long time I was depressed.

"My brother is a psychiatrist in New York, and he did a lot to see me through. He helped me to turn my anger and grief into a positive force, by becoming a patient advocate."

Harry looked at the earnest face and for a second he thought he saw weariness in her eyes. But then she drew in a breath, and went on.

"I began to counsel patients and their families. I used my skills from family law, but I also used my experiences as the mother of a patient who died. That's what I've been doing for fifteen years. I like to think I've helped people."

Irene Capek then looked straight at Harry. "I've seen a lot of doctors. I've seen some noble and some selfish, some clumsy and some skillful. I've seen doctors so callous I wanted to hit them, and doctors so compassionate I wanted to embrace them. I've stored a lot of impressions. Sometimes I've shared them with Sanford and his protégés." She put her hands in her lap, and crossed them gracefully.

"Doctors think they provide high quality care, and most of them do know the right drugs and doses. They're often obtuse at picking up how their patients feel about illnesses and symptoms. You know, how patients feel, how they react, has no correlation with how severe the disease."

"I've seen some studies on that," remarked Harry. "That's part of the quest for quality going on now in medical circles."

"Doctors really don't know the components of quality," Irene Capek responded. "I'm impressed with their willingness to share ideas, but they don't always know best. I believe patients should decide on the desirability of medical procedures. What studies show may work the best is often not what patients want.

"Indeed, I have seen reports showing that doctors pick surgery less frequently for themselves and their families than they recommend to their patients. They prescribe based on some vaguely held notion of quality, but when they or their loved ones are the patients, they become more conservative."

Harry leaned forward, nodding understandingly. "Yes, I know what you mean. I saw a paper recently that dealt with patients taking medicine to dissolve blood clots in the legs. The medicine is very effective in preventing swollen legs afterward, but in rare cases a patient may have a stroke. The study involved asking doctors what they recommended, and comparing their patients' preferences. The doctors overwhelmingly urged taking the medicine, because swollen legs after blood clots are common, and strokes are rare.

"Patients didn't see it that way. They would put up with the risk of swollen legs, rather than the hazard of a major stroke, even though the stroke occurred very rarely."

"I'm not acquainted with that study," Irene Capek commented, "but I'm not surprised to hear of it.

"In business, politics, and most areas of our society, success depends on communicating, team work, educating those involved. Doctors are taught that medical success depends totally on their own energies. That's a fallacy."

She leaned forward. "The best surgeon in the world can't get good results if the person who washes the linen for the operating room is careless."

Harry decided to change the subject. "I would imagine with the advent of managed care and for-profit health plans, you're seeing an increased demand for your services."

Irene Capek's face flushed. "Yes," she said emphatically. "I'm sympathetic to doctors and their patients, though I think both groups have brought some of these problems on themselves. The doctors have had years to see this coming. Why couldn't they have been willing to come together and collaborate? Individualism is going to be the ruin of your profession, Dr. Humbleton."

"What do you do for your clients?" asked Harry.

"I teach patients to bargain for more time. Health plans want physicians to do more, but give them less time to do it. I refer clients to doctors who use nurses and educators to help educate and communicate. Nurses are willing to spend time, and they're better at teaching patients.

"Doctors resist giving authority to nurses or social workers. In a futile attempt to maintain overall control, they're losing what patients really need from their doctors, their best informed judgment."

"You're saying that doctors could spend more time with patients if they used nurses and educators?" asked Harry. "I don't think I agree. The doctor extenders are there to increase the number of patients the doctors see."

Irene Capek uncrossed her hands, and looked upward toward the ceiling, trying to think of how to phrase her response. "No. I'm saying that doctors should spend their time learning about their patients, seeing how they respond. They need to synthesize. That's a complex function, and takes time. That's why they can multiply their healing by having staff who are extensions of themselves, but they need to spend time with the patients."

She went on. "I urge my clients to write down questions. Patients who show up with laundry lists of complaints annoy doctors, but I see it differently. It's helpful to organize one's thoughts before an important meeting. When patients bring up concerns in a succinct way, it's actually easier for the doctors to reassure them."

Irene Capek rose and began to walk around the office. Harry imagined her in a class or courtroom. She went on. "Furthermore, patients who organize themselves before- hand are actually saving the doctor and staff time in get- ting background. Medical students are taught to take a directed history, and avoid open-ended questions. But hurrying disrupts healing. In olden days doctors only saw a few patients in a work day, and had time to comfort them. Our modern technologic approach to care doesn't respect that.

"Caring for patients nowadays is more complex than it used to be. When I was a little girl in Europe, doctors pre- scribed hot baths and lozenges. Here in contemporary America, they recommend x-rays and tests, then order expensive drugs.

"Patients in turn have come to expect perfection from their doctors. They play into doctors' vanity, and then sue the doctors when they don't get what they want."

Harry decided to avoid interrupting. She continued. "Too many doctors are vain about their own expertise. Experts don't like to admit they are still learning. They're afraid to appear vulnerable or uncertain. But I tell you patients need that in doctors. That's how they relate to doctors. They have to be able to see their doctors as capa- ble yet vulnerable. They have to share certain experiences. Most of us won't open ourselves to a god.

"I'd like to help doctors see they're victims of what I call the special person syndrome. They are special, but not in the way they think. Like professional athletes and enter- tainers, they think that because of their particular talent, they deserve special treatment by others. That's not the way it should be. The doctors' desire for distance cripples their ability to heal."

Harry felt annoyed. He hadn't come here to be told how egotistical members of his profession were. "Wait a minute," he said, "Doctors are as well meaning and sincere as anyone else, and usually a lot more giving."

Irene Capek replied, "I don't say these things to insult your profession. As I said earlier, my brother that I love with all my heart, is a physician. I greatly respect the doctors I see in my work. Indeed, my reason for talking with you today is that I see myself helping nurture that human side you doctors do possess, to help it warm your souls. If you're helped, so are we patients.

"Looking after the sick is one of the highest callings to which a human can aspire. Because it's difficult, because doctors try to work as the captain of their little ships, they risk losing the very bonds that connect them to their patients, and their own humanity."

She stopped, and asked Harry, "Would you like some tea, or perhaps a soda? The discussion is getting intense."

"That's all right," Harry responded.

"I also have to get my clients to resist the compulsion to press the doctor for treatment. In our culture there's an unwritten rule that says unless one comes out of a medical encounter with a prescription, one hasn't been helped. All medicines have risks, and I want my clients to understand that often the best prescription is not for a pill."

"I wish I could get some of my patients to understand that," said Harry. "Especially when the winter viral season comes and antibiotic mania hits everyone.

"From your vantage point, do you have ideas on how doctors should change?"

"I'm not dogmatic enough to take on that task," laughed Irene Capek. "But if I were pressed for a few suggestions in this era of health plans and corporate medicine, I'd suggest doctors form large groups, and agree to take on the care of large numbers of patients. I'd try to get them to see that to meet contemporary demands for quality and flexibility, all of us must work together. Because we Europeans have lived for centuries crowded together we've had to learn a certain give and take that Americans haven't had to consider."

She stopped and breathed, carried away by the earnestness of her own cause. "I don't know if I would recommend America organize its care system like they do in Europe. Here we put ability to choose as one of our highest values. Europeans aren't so obsessed with freedom of choice. But you know one's values get filtered by one's perceptions. Let me just say that like the mythical cowboys, doctors lead isolated lives. And they pay a price. Reduce the isolation, and the personal cost drops."

The telephone on her desk rang. Irene Capek walked over to it. She pushed her hair away to get the receiver to her ear. Her mood changed abruptly. She smiled, and her voice became almost musical. "That's wonderful, my love," she said. "I'll be counting the minutes. See you at twelve."

She's flirting, thought Harry.

His eyebrows rose, and Irene Capek noticed him. "That was my husband. He has a business appointment this morning, and promised to take me to lunch afterward. We do this at least once a week. I'd invite you to join us, but we often play a little game in which we make believe we're courting each other. I plan to charm him. He will try to captivate me. Isn't that silly? But it's so much fun." A grin spread across her face.

"Mrs. Capek, I'm sure he'll love it," answered Harry.

"Please take my best wishes to Sanford," she said, walking out in front of the desk. "I'm very fond of him. And please call me again if anything I've said raises further questions." She extended her right hand.

"I'll be glad to," said Harry, as he took her hand in his. He felt her squeeze, as if to solidify her message before they parted. As he walked out he mused on Irene Capek's comments: The special person syndrome, thinking because one has a talent, he should therefore always get his way.

*    *    *    *    *

# Chapter 13.

# *Pursuing Passion*

**As** he drove home from the office that evening, Harry kept thinking about Nancy Rudolph and Irene Capek. He compared his relationship with Carol. He knew they loved each other, but he certainly didn't feel they enjoyed Nancy's and Ted's passion or the Capeks' romance. He wasn't sure exactly why. He was reluctant to bring it up at home, because it could lead to an argument, and Harry hated arguments.

Wouldn't it be wonderful for him and Carol to take off and go bicycle riding on a warm spring evening? Wouldn't it be fun to take Carol to lunch occasionally and court her? Even if they had known each other for ten years.

When he arrived home, Carol was in the kitchen, shredding lettuce for a salad. He gave her a peck on the cheek and put his coat on a chair in the living room. He went back into the kitchen and grabbed her, pulling her to him for a big hug and kiss. He ran his arms up and down her back to feel how good she was to touch.

She seemed to stiffen. He reacted by loosening his embrace, and said, "Today I had a meeting with an elderly lady who's a patient advocate. She's sixty-five, and has been married, I'm guessing, forty years. She and her husband have lunch together every week and make believe they are courting each other.

"Positively old worldly," responded Carol.

"Last week, I was introduced to the Director of Nursing at Northside hospital. We were talking about restructuring nursing education, but she mentioned she had to run off to meet her husband for a late afternoon bicycle ride. I was struck by how she looked forward to it."

"I hope they don't get hit by a car," Carol said sarcastically.

Harry came back, "I don't mean you have to run out and buy a bicycle. It was just that I was struck by how she anticipated being with her husband. She seemed to be looking forward to meeting him, and I sensed she had more on her mind than bicycling.

"The older lady is a Czech immigrant, an attorney who's a patient advocate. She must be at least sixty-five years old.

"Her husband happened to call while I was with her. She began to flirt with him over the telephone. She was grinning like an adolescent when she hung up."

Harry paused and went to the refrigerator. He took out a can of soda and popped the top. "Sometimes I get so pre-occupied with my practice and all my commitments to the medical profession that I take you and Katie for granted. I saw this lady today, and maybe because she and her husband are quite a bit older than we are, I had a twinge of jealousy. She seemed so much to be looking forward to being with him. It was romantic

"And I had the same feeling the other day hearing about the middle aged couple going bicycling together. It was simple, but she acted like it was passionate."

"Not exactly an invitation to a tryst," said Carol. "Harry, I've felt lonely many times over the years. It isn't that I resent your interest in medicine. I'm glad to see you have such a passion for your work.

"It's just that you're preoccupied. It's as though you're somewhere else. I wonder if there'll ever be room for me. I'd like to be the number one priority in your life, and when I see that I'm not, then I get angry.

"You're good to me, and I know you're a good father to Katie. For you, medicine is serious business. There doesn't seem to be much time for fun when you're a doctor. Or when you're married to a doctor."

Carol looked matter of factly at Harry and continued. "So, I've developed a parallel life over the years. Particularly now that Katie doesn't need me every hour of the day, I've started to wonder what I'll do next. She still seems small, but it won't be long before she'll start college. I worry about the empty nest syndrome. You have your profession. What's in store for me?

"I gave up nursing when Katie was born, and I really don't think I want to go back to it. I don't know what to do next. Sometimes I feel resentful."

"Do you still love me?" he asked her.

"Of course. That's never been in question. It's just that I'm afraid if I rely on you, I'll be disappointed. Many times I've waited for you to come home, desperately wanting an adult to talk with. But you were at the hospital with someone who was sick. I'd already be asleep by the time you came to bed. How was I supposed to have a passionate relationship with a man who had a mistress — his profession?"

"I know. I wasn't intentionally slighting you, but I was trying to be a great doctor. I thought the way to win your love was by being an expert physician. I kept telling myself I was doing it for you and Katie, but I was doing it for myself. Now I want to change things between us. I want to work together."

Carol turned to the stove and put a cup of pasta noodles in a pan of boiling water. "I don't know if I can change like that," she said. "I'm afraid of being let down."

"We've had a successful partnership. You made a success of your practice, and I'm doing okay raising Katie. You've been a good father. I always felt that I pushed you to give us time."

"I didn't have to be pushed," he retorted. "Being a father has been one of the greatest experiences of my life. I don't like you to imply I only spend time at home because you pressure me."

Carol wiped her hands on her apron, and looked up at Harry. "All right," she conceded. "It's just that I've developed a separate existence. I'm hesitant to give it up. Suppose you revert back? Like an alcoholic who falls off the wagon?"

"I understand," said Harry. "What do we have to do to change this? I'm saying I want to put our relationship first, to make it my highest priority. Do you believe me?"

"I do believe you. I know you're sincere. It's just that what if the siren song is still out there and starts to play again. Will you see the temptation? Will I be attractive enough to compete?"

"Lets start by committing to going out one evening every week, plus one whole day together every weekend." he said. "What do you have to lose?"

"That's a pretty low risk proposition," she said, tentatively.

"Why can't we start tonight? It's Friday. Lets get a baby sitter for Katie. I can grab a sweater, and we can go out for an Italian dinner. With red checkered table-cloths, and candles in Chianti bottles, and violins," he added enthusiastically.

"You want the whole romantic ambiance," she laughed. "Harry, you are so predictable."

"Hey, being a solid citizen is my stock in trade. There are many women who would like having a man as predictable as I am."

"Lets just say it's one of your compensating qualities," she smiled.

"Not one of my endearing qualities?" Harry raised his eyebrows indignantly.

"Okay, endearing."

"You may experience more of my endearing qualities this evening."

"I can hardly wait." She rubbed her index finger over the back of his hand.

That night, after dinner and a bottle of Chianti, the Humbletons returned home. As he was falling asleep, Harry whispered, "I do love you. I feel lucky to have you."

"You doctors think you do all the healing. We women have been supporting men's spirits since time began. We don't have certificates or diplomas, but we're very skilled healers. Spouses are supposed to heal each other. That's part of the plan." Then she dozed off.

Harry dreamed the same dream again that night. Only this time he and Carol were together on the side of the table, and she stood aside to let Harry pull the string. It straightened out and glided straight toward him, without any effort.

When he awoke the next morning Harry was drowsy, but he thought: spouses are to heal each other. That's part of the plan.

*      *      *      *      *

# Chapter 14.

# Back to the Mentor

That day Harry received a telephone call from Sanford Hayworth. "I thought it might be time about now for the two of us to get together again," he said. "You've had quite a group of mentors the past weeks. I want to hear your thoughts. Are you free for lunch next Friday?"

"Let me look at the calendar," said Harry. "No problem. No committees, no task forces, no boards that day. Where shall we meet?"

"Come by my office, and I'll get a couple of sandwiches from the deli. That way it'll be quieter for us."

"I'll be there," said Harry, and he penciled the date in his notebook.

Friday found the two physicians amidst pickles and potato salad. Hayworth reached for a plastic envelope of mustard and started talking. "I wanted to help you tell the difference between healing and curing. Remember when we started to discuss how frustrated you felt. I said you're already a healer?"

"Yes, but now I see it more clearly," said Harry. "Medical practice is actually quite abstract. Physicians' healing skills come out in subtle ways."

"When you think about it, prescribing a medicine or doing a procedure, are relatively straightforward," said Hayworth as he laid a lettuce leaf on a piece of rye bread. "To do it so that healing takes place is much more complex. Healing depends on the personality of the healer, as well as the personality of the patient. It depends on his or her self-esteem and confidence.

"Healing always involves compassion. Compassion tries to lessen pain. Patients are in pain of one form or another. That's why physicians are expected to be more compassionate than architects, lawyers, or other professionals."

Hayworth picked up a half sandwich and paused before he put it into his mouth. "Compassion certainly exists in other professionals. We doctors shouldn't think we have a monopoly on it. It's just that people who are sick have an added vulnerability. That's where our responsibilities lie, and really it's where our value to others resides.

"Harry, you have the qualities of the healer. To energize that healing spirit didn't require any major change in values. It did, though, need some changes in attitude. My hope was that by meeting these various people you could understand yourself a little better."

"So I have the power inside myself." Harry felt complimented.

"Pretty much," said the older doctor. "Practicing medicine can be enlivening and enriching. It can also be stressful and enervating. People who are sick aren't at their best. There are a lot of forces at work in our culture to distort values and turn people into objects.

"With health plans squeezing us to cut costs, malpractice lawyers lurking in the record room, and confused patients making conflicting demands, doctors have good reasons to feel stressed. The profession will straighten out and survive, because people need doctors. But it's tough right now.

"It takes maturity to sort out the real reasons for continuing practicing. I've been fortunate enough in the odyssey of my own life to be conscious of my own growth. I've watched colleagues who exhibit one or another of these graces we've talked about. The point is these qualities are what separate the healer from the body technician."

Hayworth bit into his sandwich. "It gives me pleasure when I get a chance to work with young physicians like you. And you know the best part is you might just pass these ideas on to other doctors who come after you."

\*      \*      \*      \*      \*

# Chapter 15.

# *Epilogue*

Harry made sure he kept in touch with Sanford Hayworth over the next months. He found that Leslie Ladd, Len Spector, Charlie Sharp, Bill Stokes, and Don Walters often showed up at their meetings. He came to see that he was just one in a chain of people the older doctor had influenced.

He felt proud to be in the group. Not only were they top notch physicians, they were enjoyable humans. What they seemed to share the most, however, was a sense of humor. Whether it was Leslie Ladd using her eyes to listen, or Don Walters talking about saying good-bye to patients, all epitomized some virtue he admired.

Certainly they weren't any more prominent or wealthy than the rest of his colleagues. But they did seem to be surviving, and even prospering. They had their ups and downs. Some had failed marriages. Some had major professional disappointments. But they showed a resiliency Harry admired. He decided that had to be a gift, along with intelligence, or dexterity. And it might be the most valuable in these changing times.

His own practice stabilized. The patients weren't any different from before, but he saw them as fellow humans struggling with the pains of being alive. The practice hadn't changed, he had.

He joined a multi-specialty medical group, so that he could manage his work hours better. He was pleased to find his patients understood and were considerate of his feelings. All he had to do was let them know, to share with them. He felt his practice cost less energy this way. He was able to get home for dinner on time and not feel as tired as he had.

Carol was more attractive to him than ever before. The two of them began for the first time to get to know one another. They were taking steps, even though they were tentative. Could they become lovers? Could they discover how to play together, and how to nurture each other? It would take lots of attention, and work, but he was optimistic. Spouses healing each other, that was her expression. And Harry made sure that every day, regardless of how busy he was, he took time out for healing.

*     *     *     *     *